The Nursing Career Almanac

A Roadmap to the Specialty of Your Dreams!

Mitch LaFleur DNP, RN-BC

This book is written as a source of information only. The information in this book should certainly not be a substitute for on-the-ground mentorship and guidance.

FIRST EDITION

ISBN 9798854058049

To Mom, Dad, Michelle, and Natalie. Your example, guidance, support, and love have allowed me to reach personal and professional heights I never imagined were possible. To Sadie for rescuing me. And to all the nurse managers who allowed me to join your team.

CONTENTS

ACKNOWLEDGMENTS

So many people have helped shape my experiences as a registered nurse, and whether they know it or not, they have profoundly impacted my professional career and life. One or two pages could never do each justice, but I will try my best here now. However, before acknowledging the special individuals who have foundationally helped me on my journey, I would be remiss if I didn't take a moment to recognize each of the four and half million nurses in the United States. I am in awe of you, even if we have never met.

To Mom and Dad, even the most eloquent words could never express my gratitude for your love, sacrifice, and dedication to my success. Your daily actions speak volumes, and I – and the world – am better for them. Thank you for trusting me. For allowing me to find my own path, even though it took me far from home. Knowing that your love was unconditional has helped me through some of the hardest moments of my life.

Michelle, you are my rock and my hero. The bond we have is something I will never take for granted. Thank you for standing up for me when I couldn't stand up for myself. And for believing in me when I was filled with doubt. Here's to a lifetime more of tripping over curbs as we merrily exit buildings, riding jazzy's into Walmart, and being 'set up' by wandering musicians kind enough to give us a ride home.

To Aunt Dee, for so completely and so genuinely appreciating the person I am. You have a way of making people feel truly seen, including me. Thank you for sharing in that conversation while you visited me in Wrightsville Beach. I am forever changed because of it.

Chasz, you helped raise me; I am grateful we met in front of Rachel's house all those years ago. And Bob, my cheeks never hurt so much from the laughter you constantly brought into my life; thank you. To Craig & Jeannine, I have no doubt that the only reason I stopped at Temple was to meet you both. Our friendship transcends time and space. To Jesse & Ian, for the years of smiles, surfing, and shenanigans. I always felt the love, even though we were too manly to say it.

And finally, to Ray. Thank you for taking me under your wing as a new graduate nurse [in a busy Emergency Department] with no idea what I was doing. It is a direct reflection of you that I have had any success in this profession.

i

INTRODUCTION

Welcome to *The Nursing Career Almanac*—an insightful compendium of the vast array of opportunities within the nursing profession. Whether you are an aspiring nurse or a seasoned professional, this book will be your guiding light as you embark on or seek a [new] pathway in this wonderful profession. I extend my warmest invitation to journey through these pages and embrace the wide-reaching tapestry of nursing specialties. May it empower you to make informed choices about your professional future and fill you with enthusiasm, curiosity, and a sense of adventure.

As you take a deep dive into the pages that follow, you will find a catalog of 86 nursing specialties, aiming to shed light on the known and lesser-known paths that nurses can specialize in. By gaining insights into various nursing opportunities, you will expand your knowledge and be given the keys (not literally) to unlock doors – and possibilities - that may have previously remained hidden. Your discovery of these paths can be transformative, leading you to realize your niche in the world of nursing while also reinforcing your commitment to making a difference in the lives of others.

This book is by no means a list of every possible nursing specialty or career path (maybe I'll get there with subsequent editions…). However, it is a start, and you should be proud of yourself for taking the first - or next - step toward finding your true nursing passion. I can assure you that if you look close enough, the specialty of your dreams awaits!

Mahalo,
Mitch LaFleur DNP, RN-BC
Author of *The Nursing Career Almanac*
(… and an RN who wished he had this book 'back in the day'.)

THE NURSING CAREER ALMANAC

PART I:

CLINICAL SPECIALTIES

| Medical-Surgical Nursing |

Medical-Surgical Nursing, also known as Med-Surg Nursing, is a broad specialty that focuses on providing care to adult patients with various medical and surgical conditions. Medical-Surgical nurses work in hospitals, clinics, ambulatory care centers, or specialty units. They are responsible for managing and coordinating the overall care of patients, addressing acute and chronic conditions, promoting recovery, and preventing complications.

A Day in the Life
A typical day in the life of a Medical-Surgical Nurse may involve:

1. Conducting patient assessments, including reviewing medical history, vital signs, symptoms, and laboratory results, to develop a comprehensive care plan.

2. Administering medications, treatments, and therapies as prescribed, monitoring patient response, and managing any potential side effects or complications.

3. Assisting with diagnostic tests and procedures, such as blood draws, imaging scans, or surgical interventions, and providing pre- and post-procedure care.

4. Monitoring patients' condition, including vital signs, pain levels, and response to treatment, and promptly reporting any changes or concerns to the healthcare team.

5. Collaborating with the interdisciplinary team, including physicians, surgeons, pharmacists, and other healthcare professionals, to provide coordinated care and ensure continuity of treatment.

6. Educating patients and their families about their conditions, treatments, medications, self-care techniques, and potential lifestyle modifications.

7. Assisting with wound care, including dressing changes, wound assessments, and educating patients on wound healing and prevention of complications.

8. Supporting patients and families emotionally, addressing their concerns, providing comfort, and promoting a therapeutic and compassionate environment.

9. Facilitating patient discharge planning, ensuring appropriate follow-up care, coordinating referrals to specialists, and providing education on post-discharge instructions and self-management.

10. Engaging in ongoing education and professional development to stay updated on the latest advancements in medical-surgical nursing, evidence-based practices, and patient care management.

Degree(s) Required

To become a medical-surgical nurse, you need to earn a degree in nursing. The two common degree paths are an Associate Degree in Nursing (ADN) or a Bachelor of Science in Nursing (BSN). However, some employers may prefer or require a BSN for medical-surgical nursing positions due to the comprehensive knowledge and critical thinking skills gained.

Salary

$66,640 - $110,930

Specialty Certifications Available or Needed

Certification in medical-surgical nursing can demonstrate specialized knowledge and competence. The Medical-Surgical Nursing Certification Board (MSNCB) offers the Certified Medical-Surgical Registered Nurse (CMSRN) credential. Eligibility for the CMSRN certification typically requires a combination of education, clinical experience, and the successful completion of an exam.

Job Requirements

Medical-Surgical Nursing requires a strong foundation in nursing practice and additional knowledge and skills related to the care of adult patients with various medical and surgical conditions. Job requirements may include:

1. Proficiency in assessing and managing patients with acute and chronic medical conditions, as well as those who have undergone surgical interventions.
2. Knowledge of common medical-surgical conditions, such as cardiovascular diseases, respiratory disorders, gastrointestinal disorders, renal conditions, and endocrine disorders.
3. Competence in administering medications and treatments specific to medical-surgical patients, understanding potential side effects, drug interactions, and monitoring patient response.
4. Familiarity with surgical interventions, pre-operative and post-operative care, wound management, and surgical complications.
5. Effective communication and interpersonal skills to collaborate with the interdisciplinary team, provide education to patients and families, and support patients emotionally.
6. Proficiency in documentation and record-keeping, ensuring accurate and complete documentation of patient assessments, care plans, interventions, and responses.
7. Ability to prioritize and manage multiple patients, handle emergencies,

and make critical decisions in fast-paced and dynamic environments.

8. Collaboration with the healthcare team, including physicians, surgeons, pharmacists, and other healthcare professionals, to ensure coordinated and comprehensive care for patients.

Miscellaneous Information You Should Know

To enter the Medical-Surgical Nursing specialty, you may consider the following:

1. Gain clinical experience in various areas: Acquire experience in medical-surgical units, hospitals, or clinics to develop a foundation in managing adult patients with diverse medical and surgical conditions. This experience will help you build clinical skills, critical thinking abilities, and time management skills.

2. Pursue additional education or certifications in medical-surgical nursing: Consider attending workshops, seminars, or specialized training programs in medical-surgical nursing to enhance your knowledge and skills. These programs can provide education on common medical-surgical conditions, surgical interventions, wound care, and evidence-based practices in medical-surgical nursing.

3. Develop effective communication skills: Effective communication is crucial in medical-surgical nursing to interact with patients, families, and the healthcare team. Enhance your ability to provide education, support, and empathetic care to patients and their families.

4. Stay updated with evidence-based practices: Keep yourself informed about current research, evidence-based practices, and clinical guidelines related to medical-surgical nursing. Access resources provided by professional organizations, such as the Academy of Medical-Surgical Nurses (AMSN), to stay up-to-date with emerging practices and advancements in the field.

5. Networking and professional involvement: Engage with professional organizations and communities focused on medical-surgical nursing to connect with other medical-surgical nurses, access educational resources, and stay informed about career opportunities. Participate in conferences, webinars, or local chapter meetings to expand your knowledge and network with professionals in the field.

Remember that specific requirements and preferences may vary depending on the healthcare organization, geographical location, and level of experience desired for medical-surgical nursing positions.

| Telemetry Nursing |

Telemetry Nursing is a specialized field of nursing that focuses on the monitoring and care of patients who require continuous cardiac monitoring. Telemetry Nurses are responsible for assessing, interpreting, and managing data obtained from electrocardiograms (ECGs) and other cardiac monitoring equipment. They work in a variety of healthcare settings, including hospitals, cardiac care units, telemetry units, and step-down units, where they provide vital support to patients with cardiac conditions or those requiring postoperative monitoring.

A Day in the Life

A typical day in the life of a Telemetry Nurse may involve:

1. Patient Assessment: Conducting comprehensive assessments of patients' cardiac status, including monitoring vital signs, reviewing medical history, and evaluating symptoms and response to treatment.

2. Cardiac Monitoring: Setting up and managing telemetry equipment, including placing and removing ECG leads, interpreting cardiac rhythms, and continuously monitoring patients' heart rate, rhythm, and oxygen saturation.

3. Medication Administration: Administering medications as prescribed, including cardiac medications, antiarrhythmics, anticoagulants, and other medications to manage symptoms or stabilize cardiac function.

4. Collaborative Care: Collaborating with the interdisciplinary team, including cardiologists, nurses, and other healthcare professionals, to develop and implement individualized care plans for patients, including medication adjustments, interventions, and discharge planning.

5. Emergency Response: Recognizing and responding promptly to cardiac emergencies, such as arrhythmias, cardiac arrests, or other life-threatening events. Initiating appropriate interventions, performing cardiopulmonary resuscitation (CPR), and coordinating the response team.

6. Patient Education: Providing education to patients and their families on cardiac conditions, self-care strategies, medications, and lifestyle modifications to promote heart health and prevent complications.

7. Documentation and Record-Keeping: Maintaining accurate and detailed documentation of patient assessments, vital signs, cardiac rhythms, medications administered, interventions, and response to treatment.

8. Emotional Support: Providing emotional support and reassurance to patients and their families, addressing their concerns and fears, and promoting a positive and healing environment.

9. Interpreting Diagnostic Tests: Interpreting and analyzing diagnostic tests, such as laboratory results, cardiac enzymes, and cardiac imaging

studies, to assess patients' cardiac function and response to treatment.

10. Quality Assurance and Continuous Monitoring: Participating in quality assurance activities, such as monitoring and evaluating telemetry data, identifying trends or abnormalities, and reporting any potential risks or patient safety concerns.

Degree(s) Required

To become a Telemetry Nurse, you need to earn a degree in nursing. The two common degree paths are an Associate Degree in Nursing (ADN) or a Bachelor of Science in Nursing (BSN). However, some employers or specialized cardiac care units may prefer or require a BSN due to the comprehensive knowledge and critical thinking skills gained.

Salary

$66,640 - $110,930

Specialty Certifications Available or Needed

While not required, obtaining specialty certification in Telemetry Nursing can demonstrate specialized knowledge and competency in this field. The American Association of Critical-Care Nurses (AACN) offers the Progressive Care Certified Nurse (PCCN) certification, which validates proficiency in caring for acutely ill patients, including those requiring telemetry monitoring.

Job Requirements

Telemetry Nurses require specific knowledge and skills to effectively care for patients requiring continuous cardiac monitoring. Job requirements may include:

1. Solid understanding of cardiac anatomy, physiology, and common cardiac conditions, such as arrhythmias, heart failure, myocardial infarction, and other cardiovascular disorders.

2. Proficiency in interpreting and analyzing ECG tracings and recognizing normal and abnormal cardiac rhythms, including bradycardia, tachycardia, atrial fibrillation, ventricular arrhythmias, and blocks.

3. Knowledge of cardiac medications, their indications, dosage ranges, side effects, and potential interactions. Understanding the importance of titration and monitoring of these medications based on patients' clinical status.

4. Competence in performing cardiopulmonary resuscitation (CPR), basic life support (BLS), and advanced cardiac life support (ACLS) interventions in emergency situations.

5. Familiarity with cardiac monitoring equipment, telemetry systems, and

other monitoring devices used to assess patients' cardiac status.

6. Effective communication and collaboration skills to work closely with the healthcare team, including physicians, cardiologists, and other nurses, to ensure coordinated and comprehensive patient care.

7. Strong critical thinking and decision-making skills to assess changes in patients' cardiac status, initiate appropriate interventions, and escalate care when necessary.

8. Attention to detail and accuracy in documentation and record-keeping of patient assessments, cardiac rhythms, medications administered, interventions, and response to treatment.

9. Physical stamina and the ability to work in a fast-paced environment, often with multiple patients and competing priorities.

10. Commitment to continuous learning and staying updated on advances in cardiac care, evidence-based practice guidelines, and new technologies in telemetry monitoring.

Miscellaneous Information You Should Know

To enter the Telemetry Nursing specialty, you may consider the following:

1. Gain experience in a cardiac care setting: Seek opportunities to work in cardiac care units, telemetry units, or step-down units during your nursing education or through internships and clinical rotations. This experience will provide you with exposure to cardiac patients and familiarity with telemetry monitoring.

2. Obtain advanced certifications or additional training: Consider pursuing advanced certifications, such as the Progressive Care Certified Nurse (PCCN) or Basic Life Support (BLS) and Advanced Cardiac Life Support (ACLS) certifications, to enhance your skills and demonstrate your commitment to excellence in telemetry nursing.

3. Develop strong critical thinking and assessment skills: Acquiring proficiency in interpreting ECG tracings and recognizing cardiac rhythms requires practice and ongoing learning. Focus on developing your skills in cardiac rhythm interpretation and seeking opportunities to enhance your knowledge in this area.

4. Stay updated on evidence-based practices: Keep yourself informed about current research, guidelines, and best practices related to telemetry monitoring and cardiac care.

Remember that specific requirements may vary depending on the employer, specialized cardiac care unit, or region where you plan to practice as a Telemetry Nurse.

| Critical Care Nursing |

Critical care nursing involves providing specialized care to patients with life-threatening conditions or complex medical needs. Critical care nurses work in intensive care units (ICUs), critical care units (CCUs), and other high-acuity settings. They closely monitor patients, administer medications, perform complex procedures, and collaborate with interdisciplinary teams to stabilize and support critically ill individuals.

A Day in the Life

A day in the life of a critical care nurse can be demanding and fast-paced. Some common activities include:

1. Patient Assessment: Conducting thorough assessments of patients, monitoring vital signs, and identifying any changes in the patient's condition.

2. Medication Administration: Administering medications and intravenous therapies as prescribed by the medical team.

3. Ventilator Management: Monitoring and managing mechanical ventilation for patients who require respiratory support.

4. Wound Care: Providing specialized wound care for patients with complex injuries or surgical wounds.

5. Collaboration: Working closely with the interdisciplinary medical team, including physicians, respiratory therapists, and other healthcare professionals, to develop and implement treatment plans.

6. Patient and Family Education: Educating patients and their families about their condition, treatment options, and self-care after discharge.

7. Emergency Response: Responding quickly to medical emergencies and taking appropriate actions to stabilize patients.

8. Documentation: Maintaining accurate and detailed medical records of patient assessments, treatments, and responses to interventions.

Degree(s) Required

To become a critical care nurse, you need to earn a degree in nursing. The two common degree paths are an Associate Degree in Nursing (ADN) or a Bachelor of Science in Nursing (BSN). However, many employers prefer or require a BSN for critical care nursing positions due to the complex nature of the work. Additionally, pursuing higher education, such as a Master of Science in Nursing (MSN) with a focus on critical care, can provide advanced training and leadership opportunities in this field.

Salary

$73,180 - $121,220

Specialty Certifications Available or Needed

Certification in critical care nursing can demonstrate specialized knowledge and expertise. The American Association of Critical-Care Nurses (AACN) offers various certifications for critical care nurses, including the Critical Care Registered Nurse (CCRN) certification. Eligibility for the CCRN certification typically requires a combination of education, clinical experience, and the successful completion of an exam.

Job Requirements

Critical care nursing requires strong clinical skills, critical thinking abilities, and the ability to make quick decisions in high-stress situations. Job requirements may include:

1. Proficiency in managing and monitoring critically ill patients, including advanced hemodynamic monitoring and ventilator management.
2. Skill in performing complex procedures, such as central line insertions, arterial line placements, or chest tube management.
3. Knowledge of critical care pharmacology and medication administration, including titration of vasoactive medications.
4. Ability to interpret and respond to critical lab results, diagnostic tests, and imaging studies.
5. Competence in collaborating with a multidisciplinary team to provide comprehensive care to critically ill patients.
6. Effective communication skills to interact with patients, families, and healthcare professionals in high-stress situations.

Miscellaneous Information You Should Know

To enter the critical care nursing specialty, you may consider the following:

1. Acquire experience in acute care settings: Acquiring experience in acute care settings, such as medical-surgical units, emergency departments, or step-down units, can provide a solid foundation for critical care nursing. Acute care experience helps develop skills in managing complex patients, interpreting diagnostic tests, and administering medications.
2. Pursue advanced education and certifications: Consider pursuing additional education or certifications specific to critical care nursing. This may include advanced training in critical care, such as a Master's degree or a post-master's certificate program. Obtaining certifications like the CCRN can demonstrate your commitment and competence in critical care nursing.
3. Strengthen critical thinking and decision-making skills: Critical care

nursing requires strong critical thinking abilities and the ability to make quick, evidence-based decisions. Engage in activities that enhance your critical thinking skills, such as participating in case studies, simulation exercises, or critical care nursing conferences and workshops.

4. Stay updated with evidence-based practices: Keep yourself informed about current research and evidence-based practices in critical care nursing. Access resources provided by professional organizations like the AACN or attend critical care nursing conferences to stay updated on emerging practices and advancements.

5. Develop resilience and self-care strategies: Critical care nursing can be emotionally and physically demanding. Develop self-care strategies to cope with stress, practice work-life balance, and maintain your well-being. Building resilience is essential to thrive in the challenging environment of critical care nursing.

Remember that specific requirements and preferences may vary depending on the healthcare organization, geographical location, and level of experience desired for critical care nursing positions.

| Emergency Nursing |

Emergency department nursing involves providing specialized care to patients with urgent or life-threatening conditions in the emergency department (ED) setting. Emergency department nurses work in fast-paced and high-stress environments, providing immediate assessments, interventions, and stabilization to patients across various age groups and conditions. They collaborate with interdisciplinary teams, prioritize care, and ensure timely and efficient delivery of emergency medical services.

A Day in the Life
A typical day in the life of an emergency department nurse may involve:

1. Receiving and triaging patients based on the severity of their condition and implementing the appropriate protocols for patient evaluation.
2. Conducting rapid assessments to identify patient needs, gathering pertinent medical history, and performing physical examinations.
3. Administering medications, treatments, and interventions as ordered, including starting IV lines, providing pain management, and assisting with resuscitation efforts.
4. Collaborating with physicians, physician assistants, and other healthcare professionals to develop and implement care plans.
5. Monitoring patients' vital signs, responding to changes, and providing continuous evaluation of patient status.
6. Assisting with diagnostic procedures, such as X-rays, CT scans, or ultrasounds, and interpreting the results as part of the clinical decision-making process.
7. Documenting patient assessments, interventions, and responses accurately and maintaining proper records.
8. Providing education and emotional support to patients and their families, explaining procedures, and ensuring they understand the treatment plan.
9. Participating in emergency preparedness activities, such as disaster drills and mass casualty events.
10. Collaborating with social workers, case managers, and community resources to ensure appropriate follow-up care and support.

Degree(s) Required
To become an emergency department nurse, you need to earn a degree in nursing. The two common degree paths are an Associate Degree in Nursing (ADN) or a Bachelor of Science in Nursing (BSN). However, many employers prefer or require a BSN for emergency department nursing

positions due to the complex nature of the specialty. Additionally, obtaining advanced certifications or pursuing higher education, such as a Master of Science in Nursing (MSN) or a Doctor of Nursing Practice (DNP), can provide opportunities for career advancement in emergency nursing.

Salary
$68,620 - $114,740

Specialty Certifications Available or Needed
Certification in emergency nursing can demonstrate specialized knowledge and competence in emergency care. The Board of Certification for Emergency Nursing (BCEN) offers the Certified Emergency Nurse (CEN) credential. Eligibility for the CEN certification typically requires a combination of education, clinical experience, and the successful completion of an exam.

Job Requirements
Emergency department nursing requires strong clinical skills, critical thinking abilities, and the ability to make quick decisions in high-pressure situations. Job requirements may include:

1. Proficiency in emergency assessments, including rapid physical assessments, prioritization, and recognition of life-threatening conditions.
2. Knowledge of emergency care interventions and procedures, such as cardiac resuscitation, trauma management, and emergency pharmacology.
3. Competence in triaging patients based on acuity, utilizing recognized triage systems, and ensuring timely care delivery.
4. Ability to manage and monitor multiple patients simultaneously, assessing changes in condition and responding promptly.
5. Effective communication skills to interact with patients, families, and healthcare professionals in a high-stress environment.
6. Competence in utilizing emergency equipment and technologies, such as defibrillators, ventilators, and point-of-care testing devices.
7. Understanding of emergency department protocols, policies, and regulatory requirements.
8. Skill in providing emotional support and empathy to patients and families during times of crisis.

Miscellaneous Information You Should Know
To enter the emergency department nursing specialty, you may consider the following:

1. Gain experience in acute care settings: Acquiring experience in acute

care settings, such as medical-surgical units, critical care units, or telemetry units, can provide a strong foundation for emergency nursing. Seek opportunities to work with diverse patient populations and develop skills in critical thinking, assessment, and rapid decision-making.

2. Obtain Basic Life Support (BLS) and Advanced Cardiovascular Life Support (ACLS) certifications: These certifications are commonly required for emergency nursing positions and demonstrate your competency in providing emergency cardiac care and resuscitation.

3. Pursue additional education and certifications: Consider pursuing additional education or certifications in emergency nursing. This may include attending emergency nursing courses, workshops, or pursuing advanced certifications like the Certified Emergency Nurse (CEN) credential.

4. Develop effective communication and teamwork skills: Effective communication and collaboration are critical in the emergency department. Enhance your communication skills to efficiently interact with patients, families, and the healthcare team. Develop strong teamwork skills to work effectively in interdisciplinary settings.

5. Adaptability and resilience: Emergency nursing requires adaptability and resilience to handle high-stress situations, frequent interruptions, and a fast-paced environment. Develop strategies for stress management, self-care, and maintaining work-life balance.

6. Networking and professional involvement: Engage with professional organizations like the Emergency Nurses Association (ENA) to connect with emergency nursing professionals, access educational resources, and stay informed about emerging practices and career opportunities.

Remember that specific requirements and preferences may vary depending on the healthcare organization, geographical location, and level of experience desired for emergency department nursing positions.

| Labor and Delivery Nursing |

Labor and delivery nursing, also known as obstetric nursing, is a specialized field that focuses on providing care to women during pregnancy, childbirth, and the postpartum period. Labor and delivery nurses work in hospitals, birthing centers, and maternity units, supporting women in labor, assisting with deliveries, monitoring the health of the mother and baby, and providing education and emotional support to the expectant mother and her family.

A Day in the Life

A typical day in the life of a labor and delivery nurse may involve:

1. Assessing and monitoring expectant mothers during labor, including monitoring vital signs, fetal heart rate, contractions, and cervical dilation.

2. Assisting with pain management techniques, such as positioning, relaxation exercises, breathing techniques, and administering pain medications as prescribed.

3. Providing emotional support and reassurance to the expectant mother and her family, addressing their concerns, and educating them about the labor process.

4. Assisting with the management of high-risk pregnancies and complications, such as preterm labor, preeclampsia, or fetal distress.

5. Collaborating with the healthcare team, including obstetricians, midwives, anesthesiologists, and neonatal nurses, to ensure coordinated care for the mother and baby.

6. Assisting with various delivery methods, such as vaginal deliveries, cesarean sections, or instrumental deliveries.

7. Performing newborn assessments, including Apgar scoring, and providing initial care to the newborn, including monitoring vital signs, initiating breastfeeding, and administering medications as needed.

8. Educating new mothers on postpartum care, breastfeeding techniques, newborn care, and contraception options.

9. Documenting patient assessments, interventions, and responses accurately and maintaining proper records.

10. Engaging in ongoing education and professional development to stay updated on the latest advancements in obstetric nursing, childbirth practices, and newborn care.

Degree(s) Required

To become a labor and delivery nurse, you need to earn a degree in nursing. The two common degree paths are an Associate Degree in Nursing (ADN) or a Bachelor of Science in Nursing (BSN). However, some employers may prefer or require a BSN for labor and delivery nursing positions due to the comprehensive knowledge and critical thinking skills gained.

Salary
$70,480 - $117,320

Specialty Certifications Available or Needed
Certification in obstetric nursing can demonstrate specialized knowledge and competence. The National Certification Corporation (NCC) offers the Inpatient Obstetric Nursing (RNC-OB) credential. Eligibility for the RNC-OB certification typically requires a combination of education, clinical experience, and the successful completion of an exam.

Job Requirements
Labor and delivery nursing requires a strong foundation in women's health and medical-surgical nursing skills, as well as additional knowledge and skills specific to labor and childbirth. Job requirements may include:

1. Proficiency in assessing and monitoring expectant mothers during labor, including interpreting fetal heart rate tracings, identifying signs of fetal distress, and recognizing maternal complications.
2. Knowledge of labor progression, pain management techniques, and childbirth practices, including vaginal deliveries, cesarean sections, and instrumental deliveries.
3. Competence in providing emotional support, coaching, and education to expectant mothers and their families during the labor process.
4. Understanding of common obstetric complications, such as gestational diabetes, preeclampsia, or hemorrhage, and the ability to intervene appropriately.
5. Collaboration with the healthcare team, including obstetricians, midwives, anesthesiologists, neonatal nurses, and lactation consultants, to ensure comprehensive care for the mother and baby.
6. Proficiency in newborn assessment and care, including initiating breastfeeding, administering medications, and providing postpartum education and support.
7. Effective communication skills to provide education, emotional support, and collaborate with the expectant mother, her family, and the healthcare team.
8. Proficiency in documentation and record-keeping, ensuring accurate and complete documentation of patient assessments, care plans, and interventions.

Miscellaneous Information You Should Know

To enter the labor and delivery nursing specialty, you may consider the following:

1. Gain clinical experience in relevant areas: Acquire experience in obstetric units, maternity clinics, or labor and delivery settings to develop a foundation in managing pregnancies, providing prenatal care, and supporting women during labor and childbirth.

2. Pursue additional education or certifications in obstetric nursing: Consider attending workshops, seminars, or specialized training programs in obstetric nursing to enhance your knowledge and skills. These programs can provide additional education on childbirth practices, high-risk pregnancies, fetal monitoring, and newborn care.

3. Develop effective communication and patient education skills: Effective communication is crucial in labor and delivery nursing to provide education, support, and guidance to expectant mothers and their families. Enhance your ability to communicate sensitively, provide emotional support, and adapt your communication style to meet patients' and families' needs.

4. Stay updated with evidence-based practices: Keep yourself informed about current research, evidence-based practices, and clinical guidelines related to obstetric nursing and childbirth. Access resources provided by professional organizations, such as the Association of Women's Health, Obstetric, and Neonatal Nurses (AWHONN), to stay up-to-date with emerging practices and advancements in the field.

5. Networking and professional involvement: Engage with professional organizations to connect with other labor and delivery nurses, access educational resources, and stay informed about career opportunities. Participate in conferences, webinars, or local chapter meetings to expand your knowledge and network with professionals in the field.

Remember that specific requirements and preferences may vary depending on the healthcare organization, geographical location, and level of experience desired for labor and delivery nursing positions.

| Maternal-Child Nursing |

Maternal-child nursing, also known as perinatal nursing or obstetric nursing, is a specialized field that focuses on providing care to women during pregnancy, childbirth, and the postpartum period, as well as to newborn infants. Maternal-child nurses work in hospitals, birthing centers, maternity units, or neonatal intensive care units (NICUs). They support and advocate for the health and well-being of both mother and baby, provide education, and assist with the transition to parenthood.

A Day in the Life

A typical day in the life of a maternal-child nurse may involve:

1. Assessing and monitoring pregnant women throughout their pregnancy, including prenatal visits, vital signs, fetal heart rate, and growth measurements.

2. Educating expectant mothers and their families on pregnancy, prenatal care, nutrition, exercise, childbirth education, and breastfeeding.

3. Assisting with prenatal diagnostic tests, such as ultrasounds, amniocentesis, or non-stress tests, and interpreting results.

4. Providing emotional support, counseling, and reassurance to pregnant women and their families, addressing concerns and promoting a healthy pregnancy experience.

5. Assisting with the management of high-risk pregnancies, such as gestational diabetes, preeclampsia, or multiple pregnancies, in collaboration with the healthcare team.

6. Supporting women during labor, including monitoring vital signs, cervical dilation, and fetal heart rate, providing comfort measures, and assisting with pain management techniques.

7. Assisting with various delivery methods, such as vaginal deliveries, cesarean sections, or instrumental deliveries, ensuring the safety and well-being of both mother and baby.

8. Providing immediate care to the newborn, including newborn assessments, Apgar scoring, cord clamping, initiating breastfeeding, and administering medications as needed.

9. Assisting with postpartum care, including monitoring the recovery of the mother, assessing postpartum complications, providing education on self-care, breastfeeding, and newborn care.

10. Collaborating with the healthcare team, including obstetricians, midwives, pediatricians, and lactation consultants, to ensure comprehensive care for both mother and baby.

Degree(s) Required

To become a maternal-child nurse, you need to earn a degree in nursing. The two common degree paths are an Associate Degree in Nursing (ADN) or a Bachelor of Science in Nursing (BSN). However, some employers may prefer or require a BSN for maternal-child nursing positions due to the comprehensive knowledge and critical thinking skills gained.

Salary
$70,480 - $117,320

Specialty Certifications Available or Needed
Certification in maternal-child nursing can demonstrate specialized knowledge and competence. The National Certification Corporation (NCC) offers several certifications in maternal-child health, including the Inpatient Obstetric Nursing (RNC-OB) credential, Neonatal Intensive Care Nursing (RNC-NIC) credential, or Low-Risk Neonatal Nursing (RNC-LRN) credential. Eligibility for these certifications typically requires a combination of education, clinical experience, and the successful completion of an exam.

Job Requirements
Maternal-child nursing requires a strong foundation in women's health, obstetric nursing, and neonatal care, as well as additional knowledge and skills specific to maternal-child health. Job requirements may include:

1. Proficiency in assessing and monitoring the health of pregnant women, including prenatal assessments, identifying signs of complications, and managing high-risk pregnancies.

2. Understanding of labor progression, pain management techniques, childbirth practices, and neonatal resuscitation procedures.

3. Knowledge of newborn assessments, breastfeeding support, and care of the newborn immediately after birth.

4. Competence in providing emotional support, education, and counseling to expectant mothers and their families throughout the perinatal period.

5. Collaboration with the healthcare team, including obstetricians, midwives, pediatricians, and lactation consultants, to provide coordinated care for both mother and baby.

6. Proficiency in documentation and record-keeping, ensuring accurate and complete documentation of patient assessments, care plans, interventions, and responses.

7. Effective communication and interpersonal skills to provide education, emotional support, and collaborate with the expectant mother, her family, and the healthcare team.

Miscellaneous Information You Should Know

To enter the maternal-child nursing specialty, you may consider the following:

1. Gain clinical experience in relevant areas: Acquire experience in obstetric units, maternity clinics, or labor and delivery settings to develop a foundation in managing pregnancies, providing prenatal care, and supporting women during labor and childbirth.

2. Pursue additional education or certifications in maternal-child nursing: Consider attending workshops, seminars, or specialized training programs in maternal-child nursing to enhance your knowledge and skills. These programs can provide additional education on childbirth practices, high-risk pregnancies, neonatal care, and breastfeeding support.

3. Develop effective communication and patient education skills: Effective communication is crucial in maternal-child nursing to provide education, support, and guidance to expectant mothers and their families. Enhance your ability to communicate sensitively, provide emotional support, and adapt your communication style to meet patients' and families' needs.

4. Stay updated with evidence-based practices: Keep yourself informed about current research, evidence-based practices, and clinical guidelines related to maternal-child nursing and perinatal care. Access resources provided by professional organizations, such as the Association of Women's Health, Obstetric, and Neonatal Nurses (AWHONN), to stay up-to-date with emerging practices and advancements in the field.

5. Networking and professional involvement: Engage with professional organizations to connect with other maternal-child nurses, access educational resources, and stay informed about career opportunities. Participate in conferences, webinars, or local chapter meetings to expand your knowledge and network with professionals in the field.

Remember that specific requirements and preferences may vary depending on the healthcare organization, geographical location, and level of experience desired for maternal-child nursing positions.

| Pediatric Nursing |

Pediatric nursing is a specialized field that focuses on providing healthcare to infants, children, and adolescents. Pediatric nurses play a crucial role in promoting the health and well-being of young patients, as well as managing their acute and chronic healthcare needs. They work in a variety of settings, including hospitals, pediatric clinics, schools, and community healthcare centers, collaborating with interdisciplinary teams to provide comprehensive care to pediatric patients and their families.

A Day in the Life

A typical day in the life of a pediatric nurse may involve:

1. Assessing and monitoring the physical and developmental health of pediatric patients, including growth parameters, vital signs, and behavioral cues.

2. Administering medications, vaccines, and treatments, ensuring accurate dosages and monitoring for any adverse reactions.

3. Assisting in procedures, such as venipuncture, IV insertions, and wound care, using age-appropriate techniques and providing emotional support to the child and their family.

4. Educating patients and their families about healthy lifestyle habits, growth and development milestones, and managing common pediatric conditions.

5. Collaborating with the interdisciplinary team, including physicians, pediatric specialists, social workers, and child life specialists, to develop and implement individualized care plans.

6. Providing emotional support and counseling to patients and families, addressing anxiety, fear, and the psychosocial impact of illness or hospitalization.

7. Advocating for the rights and well-being of pediatric patients, ensuring their voices are heard, and their unique needs are met.

8. Assisting families with coping strategies and resources during challenging healthcare experiences, such as chronic illness, disabilities, or end-of-life care.

9. Coordinating and facilitating pediatric healthcare services, including referrals, consultations, and follow-up care.

10. Engaging in ongoing education and professional development to stay updated on pediatric-specific healthcare practices, evidence-based guidelines, and advancements in pediatric nursing.

Degree(s) Required

To become a pediatric nurse, you need to earn a degree in nursing. The two common degree paths are an Associate Degree in Nursing (ADN) or a Bachelor of Science in Nursing (BSN). However, some employers may prefer or require a BSN for pediatric nursing positions due to the comprehensive knowledge and critical thinking skills gained.

Salary
$64,470 - $107,740

Specialty Certifications Available or Needed
Certification in pediatric nursing can demonstrate specialized knowledge and competence. The Pediatric Nursing Certification Board (PNCB) offers several certifications, including the Certified Pediatric Nurse (CPN) and the Certified Pediatric Nurse Practitioner (CPNP) credentials. Eligibility for these certifications typically requires a combination of education, clinical experience in pediatric nursing, and successful completion of an exam.

Job Requirements
Pediatric nursing requires a strong foundation in nursing practice, as well as additional knowledge and skills specific to pediatric care. Job requirements may include:

1. Proficiency in pediatric assessments, including growth and development milestones, age-appropriate vital signs, and the ability to recognize and respond to signs of pediatric emergencies.
2. Understanding of common pediatric conditions, illnesses, and their management, including respiratory infections, asthma, diabetes, and behavioral disorders.
3. Familiarity with pediatric medication administration, dosage calculations, and the ability to adapt interventions to meet the unique needs of children.
4. Effective communication and counseling skills to interact with children of different ages, as well as their families, using age-appropriate language and techniques.
5. Collaboration with the healthcare team to provide comprehensive care and ensure a holistic approach to pediatric patients' physical, emotional, and psychosocial needs.
6. Proficiency in documentation and record-keeping, ensuring accurate and thorough documentation of assessments, care plans, interventions, and patient responses.
7. Ability to provide age-appropriate education to patients and families, including health promotion, injury prevention, and self-care management.
8. Knowledge of growth and development principles, including understanding the physical, cognitive, and psychosocial changes that occur

at different stages of childhood.

9. Ability to provide emotional support, empathy, and counseling to children and families during challenging healthcare experiences, such as hospitalization or chronic illness.

10. Ability to stay updated with current research, evidence-based practices, and clinical guidelines related to pediatric nursing.

Miscellaneous Information You Should Know

To enter the pediatric nursing specialty, you may consider the following:

1. Gain clinical experience in pediatrics: Acquire experience in pediatric settings, such as pediatric units, pediatric clinics, or pediatric specialty areas, to develop a foundation in caring for children and adolescents.

2. Pursue additional education or certifications in pediatric nursing: Consider attending workshops, seminars, or specialized training programs in pediatric nursing to enhance your knowledge and skills. These programs can provide education on pediatric assessments, growth and development, family-centered care, and evidence-based practices in pediatric nursing.

3. Stay updated with evidence-based practices: Keep yourself informed about current research, evidence-based practices, and clinical guidelines related to pediatric nursing. Access resources provided by professional organizations, such as the Society of Pediatric Nurses (SPN), to stay up-to-date with emerging practices and advancements in the field.

4. Networking and professional involvement: Engage with professional organizations and communities focused on pediatric nursing to connect with other pediatric nurses, access educational resources, and stay informed about career opportunities. Participate in conferences, webinars, or local chapter meetings to expand your knowledge and network with professionals in the field.

Remember that specific requirements and preferences may vary depending on the healthcare organization, geographical location, and level of experience desired for pediatric nursing positions.

| Psychiatric Nursing |

Psychiatric nursing, also known as mental health nursing, is a specialized field that focuses on providing healthcare to individuals experiencing mental health disorders or psychiatric conditions. Psychiatric nurses play a crucial role in assessing patients' mental health, providing therapeutic interventions, administering psychiatric medications, and promoting overall well-being. They work in various settings, including hospitals, psychiatric clinics, community mental health centers, and correctional facilities, collaborating with a multidisciplinary team to support patients in their mental health journey.

A Day in the Life

A typical day in the life of a psychiatric nurse may involve:

1. Assessing Patients: Conducting comprehensive mental health assessments, including evaluating patients' mental status, identifying psychiatric symptoms, and assessing for potential risk factors.

2. Developing Treatment Plans: Collaborating with patients, their families, and the healthcare team to develop individualized treatment plans based on patients' needs, goals, and preferences.

3. Administering Medications: Administering psychiatric medications as prescribed, monitoring their effectiveness, and managing any potential side effects.

4. Providing Therapeutic Interventions: Engaging in therapeutic communication and implementing evidence-based interventions to support patients in managing their mental health challenges. This may include individual counseling, group therapy, cognitive-behavioral techniques, or crisis intervention.

5. Monitoring Patient Progress: Regularly assessing patients' response to treatment, tracking their mental health improvements, and modifying treatment plans as necessary.

6. Collaborating with the Healthcare Team: Working closely with psychiatrists, psychologists, social workers, and other mental health professionals to ensure coordinated care and holistic support for patients.

7. Educating Patients and Families: Providing psychoeducation to patients and their families about mental health conditions, treatment options, coping strategies, and self-care techniques.

8. Crisis Management: Responding to psychiatric emergencies, conducting risk assessments, and implementing appropriate crisis management interventions to ensure patient safety.

9. Documentation and Record-Keeping: Maintaining accurate and detailed documentation of patient assessments, treatment plans,

interventions, and progress.

10. Ongoing Education: Engaging in continuing education and staying updated on the latest advancements, evidence-based practices, and research in psychiatric nursing to provide the best care for patients.

Degree(s) Required

To become a psychiatric nurse, you need to earn a degree in nursing. The two common degree paths are an Associate Degree in Nursing (ADN) or a Bachelor of Science in Nursing (BSN). However, some employers may prefer or require a BSN for psychiatric nursing positions due to the comprehensive knowledge and critical thinking skills gained.

Salary

$66,640 - $110,930

Specialty Certifications Available or Needed

Certification in psychiatric nursing can demonstrate specialized knowledge and competence. The American Nurses Credentialing Center (ANCC) offers the Psychiatric-Mental Health Nurse Practitioner (PMHNP-BC) and the Psychiatric-Mental Health Registered Nurse (PMH-RN) credentials. Eligibility for these certifications typically requires a combination of education, clinical experience in psychiatric nursing, and successful completion of an exam.

Job Requirements

Psychiatric nursing requires a strong foundation in nursing practice, as well as additional knowledge and skills specific to mental health care. Job requirements may include:

1. Proficiency in conducting mental health assessments, including evaluating patients' mental status, psychiatric symptoms, and risk factors for self-harm or harm to others.

2. Knowledge of mental health disorders, psychiatric medications, and evidence-based treatment modalities, including psychotherapy techniques and psychopharmacology.

3. Understanding of therapeutic communication and counseling techniques to establish trust, build rapport, and engage patients in their treatment plans.

4. Collaboration with the healthcare team to ensure coordinated care, including attending multidisciplinary meetings, participating in treatment planning, and sharing information about patients' progress.

5. Proficiency in crisis intervention and de-escalation techniques to manage acute psychiatric emergencies.

6. Ability to provide patient and family education about mental health conditions, treatment options, and community resources.

7. Documentation and record-keeping skills, ensuring accurate and thorough documentation of patient assessments, treatment plans, interventions, and outcomes.

8. Empathy, compassion, and strong interpersonal skills to effectively support individuals experiencing mental health challenges.

9. Ability to work in a non-judgmental and culturally sensitive manner, respecting patients' diverse backgrounds and beliefs.

10. Ability to stay updated with current research, evidence-based practices, and clinical guidelines related to psychiatric nursing.

Miscellaneous Information You Should Know

To enter the psychiatric nursing specialty, you may consider the following:

1. Gain clinical experience in psychiatric settings: Acquire experience in areas such as psychiatric hospitals, community mental health centers, or outpatient clinics to develop a foundation in caring for individuals with mental health disorders.

2. Pursue additional education or certifications in psychiatric nursing: Consider attending workshops, seminars, or specialized training programs in psychiatric nursing to enhance your knowledge and skills. These programs can provide education on therapeutic interventions, psychopharmacology, crisis management, and evidence-based practices in psychiatric nursing.

3. Stay updated with evidence-based practices: Keep yourself informed about current research, evidence-based practices, and clinical guidelines related to psychiatric nursing. Access resources provided by professional organizations, such as the American Psychiatric Nurses Association (APNA), to stay up-to-date with emerging practices and advancements in the field.

4. Networking and professional involvement: Engage with professional organizations and communities focused on psychiatric nursing to connect with other psychiatric nurses, access educational resources, and stay informed about career opportunities.

Remember that specific requirements and preferences may vary depending on the healthcare organization, geographical location, and level of experience desired for psychiatric nursing positions.

| Orthopedic Nursing |

Orthopedic nursing is a specialized field that focuses on providing care to patients with musculoskeletal conditions and disorders. Orthopedic nurses work in various healthcare settings, including hospitals, orthopedic clinics, rehabilitation centers, and surgical centers. They play a crucial role in assessing, diagnosing, treating, and supporting patients with orthopedic issues, including fractures, joint replacements, spinal deformities, and musculoskeletal injuries. Orthopedic nurses provide direct patient care, assist in orthopedic surgeries, manage pain, facilitate rehabilitation, educate patients and their families, and collaborate with the interdisciplinary healthcare team.

A Day in the Life

A typical day in the life of an orthopedic nurse may involve:

1. Assessing and monitoring patients with orthopedic conditions, including performing musculoskeletal assessments, evaluating range of motion, and assessing neurovascular status.

2. Collaborating with orthopedic surgeons, physical therapists, and other healthcare professionals to develop and implement individualized treatment plans.

3. Assisting with orthopedic surgeries, such as joint replacements, fracture repairs, spinal surgeries, or corrective procedures, ensuring proper positioning, sterile technique, and instrument handling.

4. Managing post-operative care, including pain management, wound care, and monitoring for complications such as infections or deep vein thrombosis.

5. Educating patients and their families about orthopedic conditions, surgical procedures, rehabilitation exercises, and strategies for promoting healing and preventing complications.

6. Administering medications, including pain medications, muscle relaxants, and antibiotics, and monitoring their effects on patient recovery and comfort.

7. Assisting in the application and management of orthopedic devices, such as casts, splints, braces, or traction, ensuring proper fit, alignment, and patient education.

8. Facilitating physical therapy and rehabilitation for patients, coordinating therapy sessions, teaching exercises, and monitoring progress.

9. Managing patient mobility and transfers, ensuring proper body mechanics, safe ambulation, and prevention of falls or further injury.

10. Engaging in ongoing education and professional development to

stay updated on the latest advancements in orthopedic nursing, evidence-based practices, and orthopedic treatments.

Degree(s) Required

To become an orthopedic nurse, you need to earn a degree in nursing. The two common degree paths are an Associate Degree in Nursing (ADN) or a Bachelor of Science in Nursing (BSN). However, some employers may prefer or require a BSN for orthopedic nursing positions due to the comprehensive knowledge and critical thinking skills gained.

Salary

$66,640 - $110,930

Specialty Certifications Available or Needed

Certification in orthopedic nursing can demonstrate specialized knowledge and competence. The Orthopaedic Nurses Certification Board (ONCB) offers the Orthopaedic Nurse Certified (ONC) credential. Eligibility for the ONC certification typically requires a combination of education, clinical experience in orthopedic nursing, and successful completion of an exam.

Job Requirements

Orthopedic nursing requires a strong foundation in nursing practice, as well as additional knowledge and skills specific to orthopedic care. Job requirements may include:

1. Proficiency in performing musculoskeletal assessments, including knowledge of bone structure, joint function, and common orthopedic conditions.

2. Understanding of various orthopedic surgeries and procedures, including pre-operative and post-operative care, surgical asepsis, and sterile techniques.

3. Familiarity with orthopedic devices and equipment, such as casts, traction, external fixators, or orthotic devices, including proper application, care, and patient education.

4. Effective communication and patient education skills to provide comprehensive information to patients and their families about orthopedic conditions, treatment options, and post-procedure care.

5. Collaboration with the healthcare team, including orthopedic surgeons, physical therapists, occupational therapists, and social workers, to provide coordinated and patient-centered care.

6. Proficiency in documentation and record-keeping, ensuring accurate and complete documentation of patient assessments, treatment plans,

interventions, and responses.

7. Ability to adapt to a dynamic and often fast-paced environment, handle emergencies or complications related to orthopedic conditions or surgeries, and make critical decisions to ensure patient safety and well-being.

8. Knowledge of orthopedic medications, including pain management strategies, antibiotics, anti-inflammatory drugs, and medications for managing muscle spasms.

9. Ability to provide emotional support, empathy, and counseling to patients and their families during the challenges of orthopedic conditions, surgeries, and rehabilitation.

10. Ability to stay updated with current research, evidence-based practices, and clinical guidelines related to orthopedic nursing.

Miscellaneous Information You Should Know

To enter the orthopedic nursing specialty, you may consider the following:

1. Gain clinical experience in orthopedics or related areas: Acquire experience in orthopedic units, orthopedic clinics, or surgical centers to develop a foundation in managing patients with orthopedic conditions, understanding orthopedic surgeries, and assisting in post-operative care and rehabilitation.

2. Pursue additional education or certifications in orthopedic nursing: Consider attending workshops, seminars, or specialized training programs in orthopedic nursing to enhance your knowledge and skills. These programs can provide education on orthopedic assessments, surgical procedures, rehabilitation strategies, and evidence-based practices in orthopedics.

3. Keep yourself informed about current research, evidence-based practices, and clinical guidelines related to orthopedic nursing. Access resources provided by professional organizations, such as the National Association of Orthopaedic Nurses (NAON), to stay up-to-date with emerging practices and advancements in the field.

4. Networking and professional involvement: Engage with professional organizations and communities focused on orthopedic nursing to connect with other orthopedic nurses, access educational resources, and stay informed about career opportunities. Participate in conferences or local chapter meetings to expand your knowledge and network.

Remember that specific requirements may vary depending on the healthcare organization, geographical location, and experience level desired for orthopedic nursing positions.

| Ambulatory Care Nursing |

Ambulatory care nursing involves providing comprehensive healthcare services to patients in outpatient settings, such as clinics, medical offices, and ambulatory surgery centers. Ambulatory care nurses focus on managing and coordinating care for patients who do not require hospitalization, but still require medical attention, treatment, and monitoring.

A Day in the Life
A typical day in the life of an ambulatory care nurse may involve:

1. Conducting patient assessments, including health history, vital signs, and medication reconciliation.

2. Assisting with minor procedures, vaccinations, and wound care.

3. Educating patients on managing chronic conditions, medication adherence, and lifestyle modifications.

4. Providing pre-operative and post-operative care for outpatient surgical procedures.

5. Administering medications and treatments as prescribed by healthcare providers.

6. Collaborating with physicians, nurse practitioners, and other healthcare team members to develop and implement care plans.

7. Facilitating patient referrals to specialty services or diagnostic tests.

8. Participating in health promotion and disease prevention programs within the community.

9. Engaging in ongoing education and professional development to stay updated on the latest advancements in ambulatory care nursing, evidence-based practices, and treatments.

10. Developing Treatment Plans: Collaborating with patients, their families, and the healthcare team to develop individualized treatment plans based on patients' needs, goals, and preferences.

Degree(s) Required
To become an ambulatory care nurse, you need to earn an Associate Degree in Nursing (ADN) or a Bachelor of Science in Nursing (BSN). Some employers may prefer or require a BSN degree for this specialty. Additionally, pursuing higher education, such as a Master of Science in Nursing (MSN), can provide opportunities for career advancement in ambulatory care nursing.

Salary
$67,210 - $113,960

Specialty Certifications Available or Needed

While certification is not mandatory to work in ambulatory care nursing, obtaining relevant certifications can demonstrate expertise and enhance career prospects. The American Nurses Credentialing Center (ANCC) offers the Ambulatory Care Nursing Certification (RN-BC) for registered nurses seeking to validate their knowledge and skills in this specialty.

Job Requirements

To work as an ambulatory care nurse, you should possess strong clinical assessment and critical thinking skills. The ability to prioritize and manage multiple patients, handle complex medical conditions, and coordinate care among healthcare professionals is crucial. Excellent communication and patient education skills are also essential, as ambulatory care nurses often educate patients about their conditions, treatments, and self-care.

Miscellaneous Information You Should Know

To enter the ambulatory care nursing specialty, you may consider the following:

1. Gain clinical experience: Acquiring experience in a variety of healthcare settings, such as medical-surgical units, clinics, or outpatient departments, can help you develop the necessary skills and knowledge for ambulatory care nursing.

2. Continuing education: Stay updated with the latest advancements and changes in ambulatory care nursing by participating in continuing education programs, attending conferences, and pursuing additional certifications or advanced degrees.

3. Networking: Building professional connections within the ambulatory care nursing field can provide valuable insights, mentorship opportunities, and potential job leads.

4. Consider joining professional organizations: Organizations like the American Academy of Ambulatory Care Nursing (AAACN) offer resources, networking opportunities, and educational materials tailored to ambulatory care nurses.

5. Familiarize yourself with electronic health record systems: Ambulatory care settings often rely heavily on electronic health record systems. Gaining proficiency in using these systems can be beneficial for managing patient information effectively.

Remember that specific requirements and preferences may vary depending on the healthcare organization, geographical location, and level of experience desired for ambulatory care nursing positions.

| Burn Care Nursing |

Burn care nursing involves providing specialized care to patients with burn injuries. Burn care nurses work in collaboration with a multidisciplinary team to assess, treat, and manage burn wounds, promote healing, and support patients' physical and emotional recovery. They play a critical role in providing wound care, administering medications, monitoring vital signs, and educating patients and their families about burn injury management.

A Day-in-the-Life

A typical day in the life of burn care nurse may involve:

1. Conducting initial assessments of burn patients, including the extent and depth of burn injuries.
2. Administering pain medications, wound dressings, and treatments to promote wound healing.
3. Monitoring patients' vital signs, fluid balance, and respiratory status closely.
4. Collaborating with a multidisciplinary team, including surgeons, wound care specialists, physical therapists, and occupational therapists, to develop and implement individualized care plans.
5. Providing emotional support and education to patients and their families on wound care, pain management, and post-discharge care.
6. Assisting in burn wound debridement and surgical procedures as needed.
7. Monitoring and managing complications such as infection, sepsis, and organ dysfunction.
8. Facilitating patient rehabilitation and working toward improving functional outcomes.
9. Participating in burn prevention and community education programs.
10. Engaging in ongoing education and professional development to stay updated on the latest advancements in burn care nursing, evidence-based practices, and resuscitation treatments.

Degree(s) Required

To become a burn care nurse, you need to earn a degree in nursing. The two common degree paths are an Associate Degree in Nursing (ADN) or a Bachelor of Science in Nursing (BSN). Some employers may prefer or require a BSN for this specialty. Additionally, pursuing higher education, such as a Master of Science in Nursing (MSN) or a Doctor of Nursing Practice (DNP), can provide opportunities for career advancement in burn care nursing.

Salary
$67,210 - $113,960

Specialty Certifications Available or Needed
While certification is not mandatory for burn care nursing, obtaining relevant certifications can demonstrate specialized knowledge and enhance career prospects. The American Burn Association (ABA) offers the Certified Burn Registered Nurse (CBRN) certification, which validates expertise in burn care nursing. Eligibility for this certification requires a specific amount of clinical experience in burn care and the successful completion of an exam.

Job Requirements
Burn care nursing requires strong clinical skills, compassion, and the ability to handle challenging and emotionally charged situations. Job requirements may include:

1. Proficiency in burn wound assessment, management, and dressing changes.
2. Knowledge of burn injury classifications, including partial-thickness and full-thickness burns.
3. Understanding of pain management techniques and the administration of analgesics.
4. Expertise in infection prevention and control measures specific to burn wounds.
5. Ability to assess and manage complications associated with burn injuries, such as inhalation injuries or fluid and electrolyte imbalances.
6. Skill in patient and family education regarding wound care, pain management, and psychosocial support.

Miscellaneous Information You Should Know
To enter the burn care nursing specialty, you may consider the following:

1. Gain experience in acute or critical care: Acquiring experience in acute care settings, such as intensive care units (ICUs) or emergency departments, can provide valuable skills in managing complex patients, monitoring vital signs, and administering medications. Burn patients often require specialized care in critical care settings.
2. Seek burn care clinical rotations or internships: Look for opportunities to participate in burn care clinical rotations or internships during your nursing education. These experiences can provide hands-on

exposure to burn care nursing and enhance your understanding of burn wound management.

3. Continual learning: Stay updated with the latest advancements in burn care nursing by attending conferences, workshops, and seminars focused on burn care. Additionally, access resources provided by organizations like the American Burn Association (ABA) to expand your knowledge and skills in this specialty.

4. Develop communication skills: Burn care nursing involves interacting with patients and their families who may be experiencing significant physical and emotional distress. Developing effective communication skills and empathy is essential to provide appropriate support and education.

5. Networking and mentorship: Connect with burn care nurses and professionals in the field through networking events, professional organizations like the American Burn Association (ABA), or online platforms. Building relationships and seeking mentorship can provide guidance and support as you pursue a career in burn care nursing.

Remember that specific requirements and preferences may vary depending on the healthcare organization, geographical location, and level of experience desired for burn care nursing positions.

| Dialysis Nursing |

Dialysis nursing involves providing specialized care to patients undergoing dialysis treatment, which is a process that helps filter waste products and excess fluids from the blood when the kidneys are unable to function properly. Dialysis nurses work closely with patients in various settings, such as dialysis centers, hospitals, or home dialysis programs. They assess patients' needs, administer dialysis treatments, monitor vital signs, educate patients and their families, and collaborate with the healthcare team to optimize patient outcomes.

A Day in the Life

A typical day in the life of a dialysis nurse may involve:

1. Preparing dialysis equipment, including machines, filters, and dialysate solutions, and ensuring they are functioning properly.
2. Reviewing patients' medical history, assessing vital signs, and collecting relevant information to determine the appropriate dialysis treatment plan.
3. Assisting patients in accessing vascular access points for dialysis, such as arteriovenous fistulas, grafts, or central venous catheters.
4. Initiating, monitoring, and discontinuing dialysis treatments, ensuring patient safety and adherence to protocols.
5. Monitoring patients during dialysis, assessing vital signs, and observing for any adverse reactions or complications.
6. Administering medications, such as heparin or erythropoietin, as prescribed to manage blood clotting or anemia.
7. Educating patients and their families about self-care practices, dietary restrictions, fluid intake monitoring, and medication management.
8. Collaborating with nephrologists, dietitians, social workers, and other healthcare professionals to develop comprehensive care plans for patients.
9. Documenting patient assessments, treatments, and outcomes accurately and maintaining proper records.

Degree(s) Required

To become a dialysis nurse, you need to earn a degree in nursing. The two common degree paths are an Associate Degree in Nursing (ADN) or a Bachelor of Science in Nursing (BSN). However, some employers may prefer or require a BSN for dialysis nursing positions due to the complex nature of the specialty. Additionally, obtaining specialized education or certifications in nephrology nursing can enhance your knowledge and skills in this field.

Salary
$64,860 - $110,260

Specialty Certifications Available or Needed

Certification in nephrology nursing can demonstrate specialized knowledge and expertise as a dialysis nurse. The Nephrology Nursing Certification Commission (NNCC) offers various certifications for nephrology nurses, including the Certified Dialysis Nurse (CDN) and Certified Nephrology Nurse (CNN) credentials. Eligibility for these certifications typically requires a combination of education, clinical experience, and the successful completion of an exam.

Job Requirements

Dialysis nursing requires strong clinical skills, attention to detail, and the ability to provide compassionate care to patients with kidney failure. Job requirements may include:

1. Proficiency in operating and troubleshooting dialysis equipment and machines.
2. Knowledge of renal anatomy and physiology, kidney disease, and dialysis treatment modalities (hemodialysis or peritoneal dialysis).
3. Competence in assessing and monitoring patients during dialysis treatments, including vital signs, fluid status, and signs of complications.
4. Skill in accessing and caring for vascular access sites, such as fistulas, grafts, or central venous catheters.
5. Ability to manage and administer medications commonly used in dialysis, such as anticoagulants or erythropoiesis-stimulating agents.
6. Effective communication skills to educate and counsel patients and their families on dialysis treatment, dietary restrictions, fluid management, and medication adherence.
7. Collaborative skills to work within a multidisciplinary team, including nephrologists, dietitians, social workers, and pharmacists, to provide comprehensive patient care.
8. Understanding of infection control protocols and adherence to strict aseptic techniques during dialysis procedures.

Miscellaneous Information You Should Know

To enter the dialysis nursing specialty, you may consider the following:

1. Gain experience in renal or dialysis settings: Acquiring experience in renal units, dialysis centers, or hospitals with specialized nephrology units can provide valuable exposure to patients with kidney disease and dialysis treatments. Seek opportunities to work directly with dialysis patients to

develop knowledge and skills specific to this population.

2. Pursue additional education or certifications: Consider pursuing specialized education or certifications in nephrology nursing, such as the Certified Dialysis Nurse (CDN) or Certified Nephrology Nurse (CNN) credentials. These certifications can enhance your expertise and demonstrate your commitment to the specialty.

3. Stay updated with advancements in dialysis treatment: Keep yourself informed about the latest research, evidence-based practices, and technologies related to dialysis treatment. Access resources provided by professional organizations like the American Nephrology Nurses Association (ANNA) and attend nephrology conferences and seminars to stay current in the field.

4. Develop strong communication and patient education skills: Effective communication and patient education are essential in dialysis nursing. Enhance your ability to explain complex concepts, provide emotional support, and educate patients and their families about dialysis treatment, self-care practices, and lifestyle modifications.

5. Networking and professional involvement: Engage with professional organizations like the American Nephrology Nurses Association (ANNA) to connect with other dialysis nurses, access educational resources, and stay informed about emerging practices and career opportunities.

Remember that specific requirements and preferences may vary depending on the healthcare organization, geographical location, and level of experience desired for dialysis nursing positions.

| Oncology Nursing |

Oncology nursing is a specialized field that focuses on providing care to patients with cancer. Oncology nurses work in various healthcare settings, including hospitals, cancer centers, outpatient clinics, and hospice facilities. They play a crucial role in assessing, diagnosing, treating, and supporting patients throughout their cancer journey. Oncology nurses provide direct patient care, administer treatments, manage symptoms, educate patients and their families, and collaborate with the interdisciplinary healthcare team.

A Day in the Life
A typical day in the life of an oncology nurse may involve:

1. Assessing and monitoring patients with cancer, including physical assessments, symptom assessments, and psychosocial evaluations.

2. Administering chemotherapy, radiation therapy, and other cancer treatments, ensuring accurate dosages, monitoring patient responses, and managing potential side effects.

3. Collaborating with oncologists, surgeons, radiation oncologists, and other healthcare professionals to develop and implement individualized treatment plans.

4. Educating patients and their families about cancer treatments, potential side effects, self-care measures, and available support resources.

5. Managing symptoms and providing supportive care to patients, such as pain management, wound care, and psychosocial support.

6. Assisting in diagnostic procedures, such as biopsies or bone marrow aspirations, and providing pre- and post-procedure care.

7. Monitoring and managing potential complications related to cancer and its treatments, such as infections, thromboembolic events, or adverse drug reactions.

8. Providing emotional support and counseling to patients and their families, addressing fears, concerns, and coping strategies related to the cancer diagnosis and treatment.

9. Participating in clinical research studies and trials, as well as providing support to patients enrolled in research protocols.

10. Engaging in ongoing education and professional development to stay updated on the latest advancements in oncology nursing, evidence-based practices, and cancer treatment modalities.

Degree(s) Required
To become an oncology nurse, you need to earn a degree in nursing. The two common degree paths are an Associate Degree in Nursing (ADN) or a Bachelor of Science in Nursing (BSN). However, some employers may

prefer or require a BSN for oncology nursing positions due to the comprehensive knowledge and critical thinking skills gained.

Salary
$70,670 - $120,690

Specialty Certifications Available or Needed
Certification in oncology nursing can demonstrate specialized knowledge and competence. The Oncology Nursing Certification Corporation (ONCC) offers several certifications for oncology nurses, including the Certified Pediatric Hematology Oncology Nurse (CPHON) and the Certified Oncology Nurse (OCN) credentials. These certifications typically require a combination of education, clinical experience in oncology nursing, and successful completion of an exam.

Job Requirements
Oncology nursing requires a strong foundation in nursing practice, as well as additional knowledge and skills specific to cancer care. Job requirements may include:

1. Proficiency in assessing and managing patients with cancer, including knowledge of cancer types, staging, treatment modalities, and potential complications.
2. Understanding of various cancer treatments, such as chemotherapy, radiation therapy, targeted therapy, immunotherapy, and hormone therapy.
3. Familiarity with common oncology procedures, including the administration of chemotherapy, management of central lines or vascular access devices, and monitoring for treatment-related toxicities.
4. Effective communication and patient education skills to provide comprehensive information to patients and their families about cancer treatments, potential side effects, and supportive care measures.
5. Collaboration with the healthcare team, including oncologists, surgeons, radiologists, pharmacists, and social workers, to provide coordinated and patient-centered care.
6. Proficiency in documentation and record-keeping, ensuring accurate and complete documentation of patient assessments, treatment plans, interventions, and responses.
7. Ability to provide emotional support, empathy, and counseling to patients and their families during the challenging and emotional journey of cancer treatment.
8. Knowledge of palliative care and end-of-life care principles, including symptom management, advanced care planning, and facilitating discussions on patient preferences and goals of care.

9. Ability to adapt to a dynamic and often fast-paced environment, handle emergencies or complications related to cancer treatments, and make critical decisions to ensure patient safety and well-being.

10. Ability to stay updated with current research, evidence-based practices, and clinical guidelines related to oncology nursing.

Miscellaneous Information You Should Know

To enter the oncology nursing specialty, you may consider the following:

1. Gain clinical experience in oncology or related areas: Acquire experience in oncology units, cancer centers, or outpatient clinics to develop a foundation in managing patients with cancer, understanding treatment modalities, and providing supportive care.

2. Pursue additional education or certifications in oncology nursing: Consider attending workshops, seminars, or specialized training programs in oncology nursing to enhance your knowledge and skills. These programs can provide education on cancer types, treatment modalities, symptom management, and evidence-based practices in oncology nursing.

3. Stay updated with evidence-based practices: Keep yourself informed about current research, evidence-based practices, and clinical guidelines related to oncology nursing. Access resources provided by professional organizations, such as the Oncology Nursing Society (ONS), to stay up-to-date with emerging practices and advancements in the field.

4. Networking and professional involvement: Engage with professional organizations and communities focused on oncology nursing to connect with other oncology nurses, access educational resources, and stay informed about career opportunities. Participate in conferences, webinars, or local chapter meetings to expand your knowledge and network with professionals in the field.

Remember that specific requirements and preferences may vary depending on the healthcare organization, geographical location, and level of experience desired for oncology nursing positions.

| Surgical Nursing |

Surgical Nursing is a specialized field of nursing that focuses on providing care to patients before, during, and after surgical procedures. Surgical nurses play a crucial role in assisting surgeons, maintaining a sterile environment, monitoring patients' vital signs, administering medications, and ensuring a safe and successful surgical experience. They work closely with the surgical team to provide optimal patient care in various surgical settings, including operating rooms, ambulatory surgery centers, and recovery units.

A Day in the Life

A typical day in the life of a Surgical Nurse may involve:

1. Preoperative Care: Assessing and preparing patients for surgery by reviewing their medical history, conducting physical assessments, and ensuring all necessary preoperative tests and procedures are completed. Providing education and emotional support to patients and their families to alleviate anxiety and answer any questions or concerns they may have.

2. Operating Room (OR) Setup: Ensuring the operating room is properly equipped, sterile, and ready for the surgical procedure. Collaborating with the surgical team to set up instruments, equipment, and supplies needed for the surgery. Adhering to strict infection control protocols to maintain a sterile environment.

3. Intraoperative Support: Assisting the surgical team during the procedure by handing instruments, maintaining the surgical field's integrity, and anticipating the surgeon's needs. Administering medications and fluids as prescribed, monitoring vital signs, and ensuring patient safety throughout the surgery.

4. Postoperative Care: Transitioning patients to the post-anesthesia care unit (PACU) or recovery room after surgery. Monitoring patients' vital signs, managing pain, assessing for complications, and ensuring a smooth recovery. Providing postoperative education to patients and their families regarding self-care, wound care, medication management, and signs of potential complications.

5. Documentation and Record-Keeping: Maintaining accurate and detailed documentation of the surgical procedure, patient assessments, medications administered, and any complications or adverse events that occur during the surgical experience. Adhering to legal and ethical standards of documentation.

6. Communication and Collaboration: Communicating effectively with the surgical team, including surgeons, anesthesiologists, and other healthcare professionals, to ensure coordinated and comprehensive care.

Participating in surgical team meetings and debriefings to review patient outcomes and discuss any concerns or improvements for future surgeries.

7. Patient Advocacy: Acting as a patient advocate by ensuring patients' rights, dignity, and privacy are respected throughout the surgical process. Advocating for patient safety and participating in quality improvement initiatives to enhance patient outcomes and minimize risks.

8. Professional Development: Engaging in ongoing professional development activities, such as attending conferences, workshops, or continuing education courses, to stay updated on advances in surgical techniques, perioperative nursing practices, and evidence-based care.

Degree(s) Required

To become a Surgical Nurse, you need to earn a degree in nursing. The two common degree paths are an Associate Degree in Nursing (ADN) or a Bachelor of Science in Nursing (BSN). However, some employers or surgical settings may prefer or require a BSN due to the comprehensive knowledge and critical thinking skills gained.

Salary

$66,640 - $110,930

Specialty Certifications Available or Needed

Certification in Surgical Nursing can demonstrate specialized knowledge and competence in this field. The Competency and Credentialing Institute (CCI) offers the Certified Perioperative Nurse (CNOR) certification, which requires meeting specific education and practice requirements and passing an examination.

Job Requirements

Surgical Nurses require specific knowledge and skills to effectively care for patients in a surgical setting. Job requirements may include:

1. Solid understanding of surgical procedures, techniques, and equipment commonly used in various surgical specialties.

2. Knowledge of aseptic techniques and infection control measures to maintain a sterile environment in the operating room.

3. Proficiency in perioperative nursing care, including preoperative assessment and preparation, intraoperative support, and postoperative care and monitoring.

4. Competence in operating room procedures, such as instrument sterilization, equipment setup, and surgical site preparation.

5. Ability to interpret and analyze diagnostic tests, laboratory results, and patient assessments to anticipate and respond to potential complications

during surgery.

6. Strong critical thinking and decision-making skills to act quickly and effectively in emergency situations or unexpected changes during surgery.

7. Excellent communication and interpersonal skills to collaborate with the surgical team, provide education to patients and their families, and maintain effective documentation and record-keeping.

8. Physical stamina and the ability to work in a fast-paced, high-pressure environment while maintaining attention to detail and accuracy.

9. Adaptability and flexibility to work with diverse patient populations, surgical specialties, and evolving surgical techniques.

10. Commitment to continuous learning and staying updated on advancements in surgical nursing, new technologies, and evidence-based practices.

Miscellaneous Information You Should Know

To enter the Surgical Nursing specialty, you may consider the following:

1. Gain experience in a surgical setting: Seek opportunities to work or gain clinical experience in surgical units or operating rooms during your nursing education or through internships and externships. This experience will provide you with a solid foundation in perioperative nursing principles and practices.

2. Obtain advanced certifications or additional training: Consider pursuing advanced certifications, such as the Certified Perioperative Nurse (CNOR) or Advanced Cardiac Life Support (ACLS), to enhance your skills and demonstrate your commitment to excellence in surgical nursing.

3. Build strong communication and teamwork skills: Effective communication and collaboration are vital in the surgical setting. Focus on developing excellent communication, teamwork, and leadership skills to work effectively with the surgical team and provide optimal patient care.

4. Attend continuing education courses and workshops: Stay updated on advancements in surgical techniques, perioperative nursing care, and patient safety by participating in continuing education activities. This will help you stay current with best practices and emerging trends in surgical nursing.

Remember that specific requirements and preferences may vary depending on the employer, surgical setting, or region where you plan to practice as a Surgical Nurse.

| Cardiac Catheterization Lab Nursing |

Cardiac Catheterization Lab Nursing, also known as Cath Lab Nursing or Interventional Cardiology Nursing, is a specialized field that focuses on providing nursing care to patients undergoing cardiac catheterization procedures. Cardiac Cath Lab Nurses work closely with cardiologists and other healthcare professionals to assist in diagnostic and interventional procedures, such as angiograms, stent placements, and balloon angioplasty. They play a crucial role in patient preparation, monitoring, and post-procedure care, ensuring the safety and well-being of patients throughout the cath lab experience.

A Day in the Life

A typical day in the life of a Cardiac Cath Lab Nurse may involve:

1. Patient Preparation: Assisting in the preparation of patients for cardiac catheterization procedures, including obtaining consent, explaining the procedure, and ensuring patient comfort. Conducting pre-procedure assessments, reviewing medical history, and verifying necessary lab work and diagnostic tests.

2. Procedure Assistance: Collaborating with the healthcare team in the cardiac cath lab during procedures. Assisting the cardiologist in guiding catheters, monitoring hemodynamic parameters, and providing necessary medications or interventions as directed.

3. Patient Monitoring: Monitoring patients throughout the procedure, including vital signs, cardiac rhythms, and oxygen saturation levels. Recognizing and responding promptly to any changes or complications that may arise.

4. Medication Administration: Administering medications as prescribed by the cardiologist, including sedatives, analgesics, and antiplatelet agents. Ensuring accurate dosage calculations, appropriate route of administration, and safe medication practices.

5. Documentation: Maintaining accurate and thorough documentation of all aspects of the procedure, including patient assessments, medication administration, hemodynamic data, and any complications or adverse events. Adhering to legal and regulatory requirements for documentation.

6. Post-Procedure Care: Providing post-procedure care to patients in the recovery area. Monitoring vital signs, assessing puncture sites, managing pain, and addressing any post-procedural complications or discomfort.

7. Patient and Family Education: Educating patients and their families about the cardiac catheterization procedure, post-procedure care, and any lifestyle modifications or medications needed for ongoing management. Addressing any questions or concerns and providing appropriate resources

and support.

8. Equipment and Supply Management: Ensuring the availability and proper functioning of equipment, supplies, and medications needed in the cardiac cath lab. Collaborating with the healthcare team to maintain a safe and efficient working environment.

9. Quality Assurance: Participating in quality assurance activities, including monitoring and reporting patient outcomes, participating in quality improvement initiatives, and adhering to evidence-based practice guidelines.

10. Professional Development: Engaging in ongoing professional development activities, attending educational workshops or conferences, and staying updated on advancements and new techniques in interventional cardiology.

Degree(s) Required

To become a Cardiac Cath Lab Nurse, you need to have a degree in nursing. The two common degree paths are an Associate Degree in Nursing (ADN) or a Bachelor of Science in Nursing (BSN). Some employers may prefer or require a BSN due to the specialized nature of the role. Additionally, having a strong foundation in cardiac nursing and critical care is beneficial.

Salary

$68,450 - $115,800

Specialty Certifications Available or Needed

While not mandatory, obtaining specialty certifications related to cardiac nursing and interventional cardiology can enhance your knowledge and skills in the field. Examples of relevant certifications include:

1. Cardiac Vascular Nursing Certification (RN-BC): Offered by the American Nurses Credentialing Center (ANCC), this certification validates your expertise in cardiac and vascular nursing, including knowledge of diagnostic and interventional procedures.

2. Critical Care Registered Nurse Certification (CCRN): Offered by the American Association of Critical-Care Nurses (AACN), this certification demonstrates proficiency in caring for critically ill patients, including those undergoing cardiac catheterization procedures.

*Obtaining these certifications can demonstrate your commitment to professional development and validate your specialized knowledge in cardiac cath lab nursing.

Job Requirements

Cardiac Cath Lab Nursing requires specific skills and qualities to provide quality care to patients undergoing interventional cardiology procedures. Job requirements may include:

1. Cardiac and Critical Care Skills: Strong understanding of cardiac anatomy, physiology, and pathophysiology, as well as critical care principles. Proficiency in recognizing and managing cardiac emergencies and complications that may arise during catheterization procedures.

2. Technical Competence: Familiarity with the equipment and technology used in the cardiac cath lab, including catheters, guidewires, imaging systems, and hemodynamic monitoring devices. Ability to operate and troubleshoot equipment as needed.

3. Critical Thinking and Decision-Making: Strong critical thinking skills to assess patient conditions, interpret diagnostic data, and make appropriate decisions in a fast-paced and dynamic environment.

4. Communication and Collaboration: Effective communication skills to collaborate with the healthcare team, including cardiologists, technologists, and other nurses. Ability to provide clear and concise instructions to patients and their families.

5. Attention to Detail: Meticulous attention to detail to ensure accurate documentation, medication administration, and adherence to safety protocols during procedures.

6. Ethical and Professional Conduct: Adherence to ethical standards and professional nursing practices, including maintaining patient confidentiality, promoting patient autonomy, and advocating for patient rights.

7. ACLS Certification: Advanced Cardiovascular Life Support (ACLS) certification is often required for Cardiac Cath Lab Nurses due to the critical nature of the procedures and potential for cardiac emergencies.

8. Licensing: Obtaining and maintaining a valid nursing license in the state where you practice. Complying with any additional licensing or credentialing requirements specific to cath lab nursing set by your employer or local regulations.

Miscellaneous Information You Should Know

To enter the Cardiac Cath Lab Nursing specialty, consider the following:

1. Critical Care or Cardiac Experience: Gaining experience in critical care or cardiac nursing can provide a strong foundation for cardiac cath lab nursing. Familiarize yourself with cardiac monitoring, invasive hemodynamic monitoring, and the management of cardiac conditions.

2. Training and Orientation: Employers typically provide comprehensive training and orientation programs for nurses entering the cardiac cath lab.

This may include didactic education, hands-on practice, and supervised clinical experiences to develop competence in cath lab procedures and patient care.

3. Continuing Education: Stay updated on advancements and best practices in cardiac catheterization and interventional cardiology through continuing education opportunities. Attend conferences, workshops, or seminars specific to cardiac nursing and interventional cardiology.

4. Professional Networking: Engage with professional organizations and networks specific to cardiac nursing or interventional cardiology. Connect with peers, attend meetings, and participate in discussions to expand your knowledge and stay informed about industry trends and opportunities.

Entering the Cardiac Cath Lab Nursing specialty requires a strong commitment to continuous learning, excellent clinical skills, and the ability to provide safe and effective care to patients undergoing cardiac catheterization procedures.

| Wound Care Nursing |

Wound Care Nursing is a specialized field of nursing that focuses on the prevention, assessment, and treatment of acute and chronic wounds. Wound Care Nurses play a vital role in promoting wound healing and preventing complications. They work closely with patients of all ages and across various healthcare settings, including hospitals, wound care centers, long-term care facilities, and home health agencies. Wound Care Nurses collaborate with healthcare teams to develop individualized care plans, provide wound assessments, select appropriate treatments, educate patients and their families, and monitor wound healing progress.

A Day in the Life

A typical day in the life of a Wound Care Nurse may involve:

1. Wound Assessment: Conducting thorough assessments of patients with acute or chronic wounds, including assessing wound characteristics, measuring wound dimensions, evaluating tissue viability, and identifying factors that may impede wound healing.

2. Treatment Planning: Collaborating with healthcare teams to develop and implement comprehensive wound care plans. This includes selecting appropriate wound dressings, therapies, and interventions based on the wound type, etiology, and patient's overall health status.

3. Wound Dressing and Management: Applying and changing wound dressings using sterile techniques. Managing and monitoring wound drainage, exudate levels, and odor control. Utilizing advanced wound care modalities such as negative pressure wound therapy (NPWT), hydrocolloid dressings, or wound vacuums as indicated.

4. Debridement: Performing or assisting with wound debridement procedures to remove necrotic tissue, foreign objects, or nonviable tissue from the wound bed. This may include sharp debridement, mechanical debridement, or enzymatic debridement.

5. Infection Control: Implementing infection prevention and control measures to minimize the risk of wound infections. This includes proper hand hygiene, use of sterile techniques, monitoring for signs of infection, and collaborating with healthcare providers for appropriate antibiotic therapy if needed.

6. Patient Education: Providing patient and family education on wound care techniques, self-care at home, and prevention of wound complications. This includes teaching proper wound dressing changes, recognizing signs of infection, promoting nutrition for wound healing, and emphasizing the importance of adherence to the treatment plan.

7. Collaborative Care: Collaborating with physicians, wound care

specialists, physical therapists, and other healthcare professionals to coordinate care and ensure optimal wound healing outcomes. Participating in interdisciplinary wound care rounds and providing input on patient progress and treatment modifications.

8. Documentation: Ensuring accurate and comprehensive documentation of wound assessments, interventions, and outcomes in the patient's medical records. Adhering to legal and ethical standards for documentation and maintaining patient privacy and confidentiality.

9. Continual Learning: Staying updated on current wound care research, evidence-based practices, and advancements in wound care technologies through professional development activities, attending conferences, and participating in wound care-specific workshops and seminars.

10. Quality Improvement: Participating in quality improvement initiatives to enhance wound care practices, develop evidence-based protocols, and improve patient outcomes.

Degree(s) Required

To become a Wound Care Nurse, you need to earn a degree in nursing. The two common degree paths are an Associate Degree in Nursing (ADN) or a Bachelor of Science in Nursing (BSN). However, some employers may prefer or require a BSN due to its comprehensive curriculum and broader range of nursing skills.

Salary

$66,640 - $110,930

Specialty Certifications Available or Needed

Obtaining specialty certification in Wound Care Nursing can validate advanced knowledge and expertise in this field. The Wound, Ostomy, and Continence Nursing Certification Board (WOCNCB) offers the Certified Wound Care Nurse (CWCN) certification, which demonstrates specialized knowledge in wound management. Additionally, the Wound, Ostomy, and Continence Nursing Certification Board (WOCNCB) offers the Certified Wound Ostomy Continence Nurse (CWOCN) certification for nurses interested in specializing in wound, ostomy, and continence care.

Job Requirements

Wound Care Nurses require specific knowledge and skills to provide effective care to patients with acute and chronic wounds. Job requirements may include:

1. Wound Assessment and Classification: Proficiency in assessing and classifying wounds based on etiology, depth, size, and tissue viability.

Knowledge of various wound types, including pressure ulcers, surgical wounds, diabetic foot ulcers, venous ulcers, and arterial ulcers.

2. Wound Dressing Selection and Application: Understanding of different types of wound dressings, their indications, and proper application techniques. Knowledge of wound healing principles and the ability to select appropriate dressings based on wound characteristics and goals of care.

3. Wound Healing Processes: Understanding the phases of wound healing, including inflammation, proliferation, and remodeling. Familiarity with factors that can impede wound healing, such as infection, poor nutrition, compromised circulation, and comorbidities.

4. Wound Debridement: Competence in various debridement techniques, including sharp debridement, mechanical debridement, autolytic debridement, enzymatic debridement, and surgical debridement. Knowledge of indications, contraindications, and techniques for each method.

5. Infection Control: Proficiency in infection prevention and control measures specific to wound care. Knowledge of signs and symptoms of wound infections, appropriate use of antimicrobial agents, and strategies for preventing infection transmission during wound care procedures.

6. Patient Education: Ability to effectively educate patients and their families on wound care techniques, signs of complications, and self-management strategies. Providing information on nutrition, hydration, and lifestyle modifications that promote wound healing.

7. Collaboration and Communication: Collaborating with physicians, wound care specialists, physical therapists, and other healthcare professionals to develop and implement comprehensive wound care plans. Effective communication and interdisciplinary teamwork are crucial.

8. Documentation: Ensuring accurate and thorough documentation of wound assessments, interventions, and outcomes in medical records. Adhering to legal and ethical standards for documentation.

9. Continual Learning: Staying updated on current research, evidence-based practices, and advancements in wound care through professional development activities, attending conferences, and participating in wound care-specific workshops and seminars.

Miscellaneous Information You Should Know

To enter the Wound Care Nursing specialty, you may consider the following:

1. Gain Clinical Experience: Seek opportunities to work in settings where you can gain exposure to patients with wounds, such as hospitals, long-term care facilities, or wound care clinics. This experience will provide a foundation for developing wound assessment and management skills.

2. Certification and Continuing Education: Pursue specialty certification in wound care nursing, such as the Certified Wound Care Nurse (CWCN) offered by the WOCNCB. Additionally, engage in continuing education activities and wound care-specific training programs to expand your knowledge and expertise in this field.

3. Networking and Professional Organizations: Connect with wound care specialists and join professional organizations such as the Wound, Ostomy, and Continence Nurses Society (WOCN) to access resources, educational opportunities, and networking events specific to wound care nursing.

4. Preceptorship and Mentorship: Seek opportunities to work with experienced Wound Care Nurses who can serve as mentors and provide guidance as you develop your wound care skills. Consider pursuing a preceptorship or mentorship program to enhance your learning experience.

5. Strong Assessment and Documentation Skills: Develop strong assessment skills, including the ability to accurately assess wound characteristics, measure wound dimensions, and document findings effectively. Attention to detail and meticulous documentation are essential in wound care nursing.

Remember that specific requirements and preferences may vary depending on the employer, healthcare facility, or wound care practice where you plan to work as a Wound Care Nurse.

| Endoscopy Nursing |

Endoscopy nursing involves providing specialized care to patients undergoing endoscopic procedures, which are minimally invasive diagnostic or therapeutic procedures used to visualize and treat conditions within the gastrointestinal (GI) tract. Endoscopy nurses work closely with gastroenterologists and other healthcare professionals in endoscopy units or procedure rooms. They assist with endoscopic procedures, monitor patients during the procedures, provide patient education, and ensure safe and effective care delivery.

A Day in the Life

A typical day in the life of an endoscopy nurse may involve:

1. Preparing the endoscopy suite, ensuring that the necessary equipment and supplies are available and properly sterilized.
2. Reviewing patients' medical history, assessing vital signs, and gathering relevant information before the procedure.
3. Educating patients about the endoscopic procedure, including its purpose, what to expect, and any necessary preparations (e.g., fasting, bowel cleansing).
4. Assisting the gastroenterologist during endoscopic procedures, such as colonoscopies, gastroscopies, or ERCPs (endoscopic retrograde cholangiopancreatography).
5. Monitoring patients' vital signs, oxygen saturation, and comfort level throughout the procedure.
6. Administering conscious sedation and monitoring patients' sedation levels and response during the procedure.
7. Assisting with specimen collection, biopsy procedures, or therapeutic interventions during the endoscopy.
8. Providing post-procedure care, monitoring patients' recovery, and ensuring their comfort and safety.
9. Educating patients and their families on post-procedure care instructions and potential complications.
10. Documenting patient assessments, procedures, medications, and any adverse events accurately.

Degree(s) Required

To become an endoscopy nurse, you need to earn a degree in nursing. The two common degree paths are an Associate Degree in Nursing (ADN) or a Bachelor of Science in Nursing (BSN). However, pursuing a BSN is increasingly preferred for endoscopy nursing positions due to the complexity of the specialty. Additionally, obtaining specialized education or certifications in gastroenterology nursing can enhance your knowledge and skills in this field.

Salary
$65,064 - $107,524

Specialty Certifications Available or Needed
Certification in gastroenterology nursing can demonstrate specialized knowledge and competence as an endoscopy nurse. The American Board of Certification for Gastroenterology Nurses (ABCGN) offers the Certified Gastroenterology Registered Nurse (CGRN) credential. Eligibility for the CGRN certification typically requires a combination of education, clinical experience, and the successful completion of an exam.

Job Requirements
Endoscopy nursing requires strong clinical skills, attention to detail, and the ability to provide compassionate care to patients undergoing endoscopic procedures. Job requirements may include:

1. Proficiency in assisting with various endoscopic procedures and interventions, including knowledge of equipment and sterile techniques.
2. Knowledge of gastrointestinal anatomy, physiology, and common GI disorders or conditions.
3. Competence in administering conscious sedation and monitoring patients' sedation levels and response.
4. Understanding of infection control practices and adherence to strict aseptic techniques during endoscopic procedures.
5. Skill in interpreting and documenting endoscopic findings and assisting with specimen collection or biopsies.
6. Effective communication skills to educate and support patients and their families throughout the endoscopy process.
7. Ability to recognize and respond to potential complications or adverse events during endoscopic procedures.
8. Collaboration with gastroenterologists and the healthcare team to provide comprehensive care to patients.

Miscellaneous Information You Should Know
To enter the endoscopy nursing specialty, you may consider the following:

1. Gain experience in procedural or gastroenterology settings: Acquiring experience in procedural areas, gastroenterology clinics, or medical-surgical units can provide a foundation for endoscopy nursing. Seek opportunities

to work with patients undergoing endoscopic procedures and develop knowledge and skills specific to this area.

2. Pursue additional education or certifications: Consider pursuing additional education or certifications in gastroenterology nursing, such as the Certified Gastroenterology Registered Nurse (CGRN) credential. These certifications can enhance your expertise and demonstrate your commitment to the specialty.

3. Develop effective communication and patient education skills: Effective communication and patient education are essential in endoscopy nursing. Enhance your ability to explain procedures, provide emotional support, and educate patients and their families about the endoscopy process, post-procedure care, and potential complications.

4. Familiarize yourself with endoscopy equipment and procedures: Gain familiarity with common endoscopy equipment, such as endoscopes, light sources, and video monitors. Stay updated on emerging technologies and advancements in endoscopy procedures by attending conferences, workshops, or webinars in the field.

5. Networking and professional involvement: Engage with professional organizations like the Society of Gastroenterology Nurses and Associates (SGNA) to connect with other endoscopy nurses, access educational resources, and stay informed about emerging practices and career opportunities.

Remember that specific requirements and preferences may vary depending on the healthcare organization, geographical location, and level of experience desired for endoscopy nursing positions.

| Infectious Disease Nursing |

Infectious disease nursing is a specialized field that focuses on the prevention, management, and treatment of infectious diseases. Infectious disease nurses work in various healthcare settings, including hospitals, clinics, public health departments, and research institutions. They play a crucial role in preventing the spread of infections, conducting assessments, providing education, administering treatments, and coordinating care for patients with infectious diseases.

A Day in the Life
A typical day in the life of an infectious disease nurse may involve:

1. Assessing and monitoring patients with infectious diseases, including evaluating symptoms, reviewing laboratory results, and determining appropriate treatment plans.
2. Administering medications, such as antibiotics or antivirals, and managing IV therapy or other specialized treatments to combat infections.
3. Educating patients and their families on infection prevention measures, including hand hygiene, proper wound care, isolation precautions, and medication adherence.
4. Collaborating with the healthcare team, including infectious disease physicians, infection preventionists, laboratory staff, and other healthcare professionals, to develop and implement infection control strategies.
5. Conducting infection control surveillance, monitoring trends, and identifying potential outbreaks or areas for improvement in infection prevention practices.
6. Participating in infection prevention and control committees, providing expertise and guidance on policies, procedures, and protocols related to infectious diseases.
7. Assisting with the coordination of diagnostic tests, interpreting results, and implementing appropriate interventions based on the findings.
8. Documenting patient assessments, interventions, and responses accurately and maintaining proper records.
9. Engaging in ongoing education and professional development to stay updated on the latest advancements in infectious disease nursing and infection prevention practices.
10. Collaborating with public health agencies or participating in community outreach programs to promote infection prevention and raise awareness about infectious diseases.

Degree(s) Required
To become an infectious disease nurse, you need to earn a degree in

nursing. The two common degree paths are an Associate Degree in Nursing (ADN) or a Bachelor of Science in Nursing (BSN). However, some employers may prefer or require a BSN for infectious disease nursing positions due to the comprehensive knowledge and critical thinking skills gained.

Salary
$66,640 - $110,930

Specialty Certifications Available or Needed
Certification in infectious disease nursing can demonstrate specialized knowledge and competence. The Certification Board of Infection Control and Epidemiology (CBIC) offers the Certification in Infection Prevention and Control (CIC) credential. Although not specific to infectious disease nursing, obtaining the CIC certification can enhance your expertise in infection prevention and control.

Job Requirements
Infectious disease nursing requires a strong foundation in medical-surgical nursing skills, as well as additional knowledge and skills specific to managing infectious diseases and implementing infection prevention strategies. Job requirements may include:

1. Proficiency in assessing and managing patients with various infectious diseases, including understanding disease transmission, clinical manifestations, diagnostic tests, and treatment options.

2. Knowledge of infection prevention and control practices, including standard precautions, isolation protocols, sterilization techniques, and outbreak management.

3. Competence in administering medications commonly used in infectious disease management, such as antibiotics, antivirals, or antifungals, while monitoring for potential adverse reactions.

4. Skill in educating patients and their families on infection prevention strategies, proper medication administration, and self-care techniques.

5. Understanding of the principles of epidemiology, surveillance, and outbreak investigation, including the ability to identify patterns, interpret data, and implement appropriate interventions.

6. Collaboration with the healthcare team, including infectious disease physicians, infection preventionists, laboratory staff, and other healthcare professionals, to provide comprehensive care and ensure effective infection control.

7. Proficiency in documentation and record-keeping, ensuring accurate and complete documentation of patient assessments, care plans, and

interventions.

Miscellaneous Information You Should Know

To enter the infectious disease nursing specialty, you may consider the following:

1. Gain clinical experience in relevant areas: Acquire experience in medical-surgical units, intensive care units, or infectious disease clinics to develop a foundation in managing patients with infectious diseases and implementing infection prevention practices.

2. Pursue additional education or certifications in infectious disease nursing: Consider attending workshops, seminars, or specialized training programs in infectious disease nursing or infection prevention and control to enhance your knowledge and skills. These programs can provide additional education on infectious diseases, diagnostic tests, antimicrobial therapy, and infection control practices.

3. Develop effective communication and patient education skills: Effective communication is crucial in infectious disease nursing to provide education, support, and guidance to patients and their families. Enhance your ability to communicate complex information in a clear and empathetic manner, adapting your communication style to patients' and families' needs and cultural backgrounds.

4. Stay updated with evidence-based practices: Keep yourself informed about current research, evidence-based practices, and clinical guidelines related to infectious disease nursing and infection prevention. Access resources provided by professional organizations, such as the Association for Professionals in Infection Control and Epidemiology (APIC), to stay up-to-date with emerging practices and advancements in the field.

5. Networking and professional involvement: Engage with professional organizations to connect with other infectious disease nurses, access educational resources, and stay informed about career opportunities. Participate in conferences, webinars, or local chapter meetings to expand your knowledge and network with professionals in the field.

Remember that specific requirements and preferences may vary depending on the healthcare organization, geographical location, and level of experience desired for infectious disease nursing positions.

| Neurology Nursing |

Neurology nursing is a specialized field that focuses on the care of patients with neurological disorders and conditions affecting the nervous system. Neurology nurses work in hospitals, clinics, neuroscience units, and rehabilitation centers. They play a crucial role in assessing, diagnosing, and managing patients with neurological conditions such as stroke, epilepsy, multiple sclerosis, Parkinson's disease, and traumatic brain injuries.

A Day in the Life

A typical day in the life of a neurology nurse may involve:

1. Conducting comprehensive neurological assessments, including evaluating patients' mental status, motor function, sensory perception, reflexes, and coordination.

2. Administering medications as prescribed, such as antiepileptic drugs, muscle relaxants, or medications to manage symptoms related to neurological conditions.

3. Monitoring patients for changes in neurological status, assessing vital signs, and promptly reporting any abnormalities or deterioration to the healthcare team.

4. Assisting with diagnostic tests and procedures, such as electroencephalograms (EEGs), magnetic resonance imaging (MRI), or lumbar punctures, and providing pre- and post-procedure care.

5. Collaborating with the interdisciplinary team, including neurologists, neurosurgeons, physical therapists, occupational therapists, and speech-language pathologists, to develop and implement individualized care plans.

6. Educating patients and their families about neurological conditions, treatment options, medication management, symptom management, and promoting self-care techniques.

7. Providing emotional support and counseling to patients and families, addressing concerns, and helping them cope with the challenges of living with neurological conditions.

8. Assisting with neurological rehabilitation programs, including physical therapy, occupational therapy, and speech therapy, to optimize functional independence and recovery.

9. Monitoring and managing potential complications associated with neurological conditions, such as seizures, aspiration, or falls.

10. Engaging in ongoing education and professional development to stay updated on the latest advancements in neurology nursing, evidence-based practices, and neurological care management.

Degree(s) Required

To become a neurology nurse, you need to earn a degree in nursing. The two common degree paths are an Associate Degree in Nursing (ADN) or a Bachelor of Science in Nursing (BSN). However, some employers may prefer or require a BSN for neurology nursing positions due to the comprehensive knowledge and critical thinking skills gained.

Salary
$66,640 - $110,930

Specialty Certifications Available or Needed
Certification in neurology nursing can demonstrate specialized knowledge and competence. The American Board of Neuroscience Nursing (ABNN) offers the Certified Neuroscience Registered Nurse (CNRN) credential. Eligibility for the CNRN certification typically requires a combination of education, clinical experience in neurology nursing, and successful completion of an exam.

Job Requirements
Neurology nursing requires a strong foundation in nursing practice, as well as additional knowledge and skills specific to neurological conditions and care. Job requirements may include:

1. Proficiency in assessing and managing patients with neurological disorders, including the ability to perform neurological examinations, interpret diagnostic tests, and recognize signs of deterioration.

2. Knowledge of common neurological conditions, such as stroke, epilepsy, multiple sclerosis, neurodegenerative disorders, and traumatic brain injuries.

3. Understanding of pharmacology related to neurological conditions, including the administration and monitoring of medications commonly used in neurology, such as antiepileptic drugs, muscle relaxants, and medications to manage spasticity or pain.

4. Familiarity with neurological rehabilitation principles and techniques, including physical therapy, occupational therapy, and speech therapy interventions.

5. Effective communication and patient education skills to provide comprehensive education to patients and their families on neurological conditions, treatment options, self-care measures, and community resources.

6. Collaboration with the healthcare team, including neurologists, neurosurgeons, therapists, and other healthcare professionals, to provide coordinated and patient-centered care.

7. Proficiency in documentation and record-keeping, ensuring accurate

and complete documentation of patient assessments, treatment plans, interventions, and responses.

8. Ability to adapt to a dynamic and challenging environment, handle emergencies or complications related to neurological conditions, and make critical decisions to ensure patient safety and well-being.

9. Cultural sensitivity and empathy to work effectively with individuals from diverse backgrounds and varying levels of neurological needs.

10. Ability to stay updated with current research, evidence-based practices, and clinical guidelines related to neurology nursing.

Miscellaneous Information You Should Know

To enter the neurology nursing specialty, you may consider the following:

1. Gain clinical experience in neurology or related areas: Acquire experience in neurology units, stroke units, epilepsy clinics, or rehabilitation centers to develop a foundation in managing patients with neurological conditions, understanding diagnostic tests, and becoming familiar with rehabilitation techniques.

2. Pursue additional education or certifications in neurology nursing: Consider attending workshops, seminars, or specialized training programs in neurology nursing to enhance your knowledge and skills. These programs can provide education on neurological conditions, assessment techniques, rehabilitation strategies, and evidence-based practices in neurology nursing.

3. Stay updated with evidence-based practices: Keep yourself informed about current research, evidence-based practices, and clinical guidelines related to neurology nursing. Access resources provided by professional organizations, such as the American Association of Neuroscience Nurses (AANN), to stay up-to-date with emerging practices and advancements in the field.

4. Networking and professional involvement: Engage with professional organizations and communities focused on neurology nursing to connect with other neurology nurses, access educational resources, and stay informed about career opportunities. Participate in conferences, webinars, or local chapter meetings to expand your knowledge and network with professionals in the field.

Remember that specific requirements and preferences may vary depending on the healthcare organization, geographical location, and level of experience desired for neurology nursing positions.

| Cardiac Rehabilitation Nursing |

Cardiac Rehabilitation Nursing is a specialized field that focuses on providing comprehensive care and support to individuals recovering from heart-related conditions or cardiac procedures. Cardiac Rehab Nurses work closely with patients and their families to develop personalized rehabilitation plans, monitor their progress, and educate them on heart-healthy lifestyles. They play a crucial role in promoting cardiovascular health, preventing complications, and empowering patients to regain optimal physical and emotional well-being.

A Day in the Life

A typical day in the life of a Cardiac Rehab Nurse may involve:

1. Patient Assessment: Conducting initial assessments to evaluate patients' cardiac health, exercise tolerance, and overall well-being. Assessing their risk factors, medical history, and lifestyle choices to develop individualized rehab plans.

2. Rehabilitation Program Design: Collaborating with the healthcare team to design and implement cardiac rehabilitation programs tailored to each patient's needs. This includes setting goals, selecting appropriate exercises, and determining the frequency and intensity of sessions.

3. Exercise Supervision: Overseeing exercise sessions and monitoring patients' vital signs, heart rhythm, blood pressure, and oxygen saturation levels during physical activity. Providing guidance, support, and modifications as needed to ensure safety and optimal progress.

4. Education and Counseling: Providing comprehensive education to patients and their families on heart disease, lifestyle modifications, medication management, stress reduction, and healthy nutrition. Offering counseling and emotional support to address their concerns and help them cope with the emotional impact of heart-related conditions.

5. Risk Factor Modification: Assisting patients in identifying and managing risk factors such as high blood pressure, cholesterol levels, diabetes, and smoking. Collaborating with the healthcare team to develop strategies for risk reduction and medication adherence.

6. Monitoring and Evaluation: Regularly assessing patients' progress and adjusting their rehabilitation plans accordingly. Utilizing outcome measures and monitoring tools to track improvements in exercise capacity, functional status, and overall cardiovascular health.

7. Interdisciplinary Collaboration: Working closely with cardiologists, physiotherapists, dietitians, psychologists, and other healthcare professionals to provide comprehensive care and ensure a holistic approach to patient recovery.

8. Documentation and Reporting: Maintaining accurate and detailed documentation of patient assessments, progress notes, exercise sessions, and education provided. Generating reports on patient outcomes and participating in quality improvement initiatives.

9. Community Outreach: Engaging in community outreach activities to promote heart health, educate the public on cardiovascular disease prevention, and raise awareness about the benefits of cardiac rehabilitation.

10. Professional Development: Staying updated on the latest research, guidelines, and advancements in cardiac rehabilitation through continuing education, attending conferences, and participating in relevant professional organizations.

Degree(s) Required

To become a Cardiac Rehab Nurse, you need to have a degree in nursing. The two common degree paths are an Associate Degree in Nursing (ADN) or a Bachelor of Science in Nursing (BSN). However, some employers may prefer or require a BSN due to the specialized nature of the role. Additionally, having a strong foundation in cardiac nursing, critical care, and exercise physiology is beneficial.

Salary

$68,450 - $115,804

Specialty Certifications Available or Needed

While not mandatory, obtaining specialty certifications related to cardiac rehabilitation can demonstrate your expertise and commitment to the field. One of the most recognized certifications is:

1. Cardiac Rehabilitation Certification (CRS): Offered by the American Association of Cardiovascular and Pulmonary Rehabilitation (AACVPR), this certification validates your knowledge and skills in the field of cardiac rehabilitation.

Obtaining the CRS certification demonstrates your proficiency in cardiac rehab principles, risk assessment, exercise prescription, patient education, and program management.

Job Requirements

Cardiac Rehab Nursing requires specific skills and qualities to provide quality care and support to patients during their recovery. Job requirements may include:

1. Cardiac and Rehabilitation Knowledge: Strong understanding of

cardiovascular anatomy, physiology, and pathophysiology, as well as principles of rehabilitation. Familiarity with evidence-based practices in cardiac rehabilitation, exercise prescription, and risk factor management.

2. Patient Education and Counseling: Excellent communication and teaching skills to provide comprehensive education to patients and their families. Ability to translate complex medical information into understandable terms and motivate patients to adopt heart-healthy lifestyles.

3. Clinical Competence: Proficiency in performing cardiac assessments, including vital signs monitoring, ECG interpretation, and risk factor assessment. Knowledge of pharmacological treatments commonly used in cardiac rehabilitation.

4. Critical Thinking and Problem-Solving: Strong critical thinking skills to assess patients' response to exercise and adapt rehabilitation plans accordingly. Ability to recognize and respond to any complications or changes in patients' condition during exercise sessions.

5. Documentation and Record Keeping: Accurate and thorough documentation skills to maintain patient records, progress notes, and outcomes data. Understanding the importance of confidentiality and adherence to legal and regulatory requirements.

6. Interpersonal Skills and Teamwork: Effective collaboration and communication skills to work as part of an interdisciplinary team. Collaborating with other healthcare professionals, patients, and their families to ensure comprehensive care and positive patient outcomes.

7. ACLS Certification: Advanced Cardiovascular Life Support (ACLS) certification may be required, as Cardiac Rehab Nurses may encounter cardiac emergencies during exercise sessions or in outpatient settings.

8. Licensing: Obtaining and maintaining a valid nursing license in the state where you practice. Complying with any additional licensing or credentialing requirements specific to cardiac rehab nursing set by your employer or local regulations.

Miscellaneous Information You Should Know

To enter the Cardiac Rehab Nursing specialty, consider the following:

1. Gain Experience in Cardiac Nursing: Building a foundation in cardiac nursing through clinical experience or employment in cardiac care units, such as cardiac step-down or critical care units, can provide valuable knowledge and skills in managing patients with heart-related conditions.

2. Continuing Education: Stay updated on advancements and best practices in cardiac rehabilitation through continuing education opportunities. Attend workshops, conferences, or seminars specific to cardiac rehabilitation nursing.

3. Network and Collaborate: Engage with professional organizations and

networks in the field of cardiac rehabilitation nursing. Participate in meetings, connect with colleagues, and stay informed about new research and trends.

4. Clinical Placement or Preceptorship: If possible, seek clinical placements or preceptorship opportunities in a cardiac rehab setting during your nursing education. This hands-on experience can provide valuable exposure to the specialty and help you develop essential skills.

Entering the Cardiac Rehabilitation Nursing specialty requires a strong passion for cardiovascular health, dedication to patient-centered care, and the ability to support individuals on their journey to recovery and improved quality of life.

| Gastroenterology Nursing |

Gastroenterology nursing is a specialized field that focuses on providing care to patients with digestive system disorders, including the gastrointestinal (GI) tract, liver, gallbladder, and pancreas. Gastroenterology nurses work in various settings, such as hospitals, clinics, endoscopy units, or outpatient facilities. They assist with diagnostic procedures, manage chronic conditions, and educate patients on GI health and disease prevention.

A Day in the Life
A typical day in the life of a gastroenterology nurse may involve:

1. Assisting with diagnostic procedures, such as endoscopies, colonoscopies, or liver biopsies, by preparing equipment, medications, and patients.
2. Providing patient education about the procedure, including bowel preparation instructions, risks, benefits, and post-procedure care.
3. Collaborating with the healthcare team to ensure patient safety and comfort during procedures.
4. Administering conscious sedation and monitoring patients' vital signs, sedation levels, and response during procedures.
5. Assisting with specimen collection, biopsy procedures, or therapeutic interventions during endoscopic procedures.
6. Assessing patients' GI symptoms, performing physical examinations, and reviewing medical history to develop individualized care plans.
7. Administering medications, such as antibiotics, antacids, or immunosuppressants, and managing potential side effects.
8. Monitoring and managing patients with chronic GI conditions, such as inflammatory bowel disease, liver disease, or gastroesophageal reflux disease.
9. Providing education to patients and their families on GI health, disease management, lifestyle modifications, and medication adherence.
10. Documenting patient assessments, interventions, and responses accurately and maintaining proper records.

Degree(s) Required
To become a gastroenterology nurse, you need to earn a degree in nursing. The two common degree paths are an Associate Degree in Nursing (ADN) or a Bachelor of Science in Nursing (BSN). However, many employers prefer or require a BSN for gastroenterology nursing positions due to the specialized knowledge and skills required. Additionally, obtaining specialized education or certifications in gastroenterology nursing can

enhance your expertise in this field.

Salary
$65,010 - $107,512

Specialty Certifications Available or Needed

Certification in gastroenterology nursing can demonstrate specialized knowledge and competence. The American Board of Certification for Gastroenterology Nurses (ABCGN) offers the Certified Gastroenterology Registered Nurse (CGRN) credential. Eligibility for the CGRN certification typically requires a combination of education, clinical experience, and the successful completion of an exam.

Job Requirements

Gastroenterology nursing requires a strong foundation in medical-surgical nursing skills, as well as additional knowledge and skills specific to GI health and disease management. Job requirements may include:

1. Proficiency in assisting with various GI diagnostic procedures, such as endoscopies, colonoscopies, or ERCPs (endoscopic retrograde cholangiopancreatography).
2. Knowledge of common GI conditions and disorders, including gastroesophageal reflux disease, inflammatory bowel disease, liver disease, or pancreatic disorders.
3. Competence in patient education regarding GI health, including lifestyle modifications, dietary recommendations, and medication management.
4. Skill in administering conscious sedation and monitoring patients during procedures, including knowledge of potential complications and interventions.
5. Understanding of infection control practices and adherence to aseptic techniques during endoscopic procedures.
6. Effective communication skills to educate and support patients and their families during the diagnostic and treatment process.
7. Collaboration with the healthcare team, including gastroenterologists, surgeons, dietitians, and other allied healthcare professionals, to provide comprehensive care.
8. Proficiency in documentation and record-keeping, ensuring accurate and complete documentation of patient encounters and procedures.

Miscellaneous Information You Should Know

To enter the gastroenterology nursing specialty, you may consider the following:

1. Gain clinical experience in relevant areas: Acquire experience in medical-surgical units, ambulatory care settings, or endoscopy units to develop a foundation in managing patients with GI conditions and assisting with endoscopic procedures.

2. Pursue additional education or certifications in gastroenterology nursing: Consider attending workshops, seminars, or specialized training programs in gastroenterology nursing to enhance your knowledge and skills. These programs can provide additional education on specific GI conditions, endoscopic techniques, and patient education strategies.

3. Develop effective communication and patient education skills: Effective communication and patient education are crucial in gastroenterology nursing. Enhance your ability to explain complex GI conditions, procedures, and treatment plans to patients and their families. Develop strategies to support patients in managing their conditions and making informed decisions.

4. Stay updated with evidence-based practices and guidelines: Keep yourself informed about current research, evidence-based practices, and clinical guidelines related to gastroenterology nursing. Access resources provided by professional organizations, such as the Society of Gastroenterology Nurses and Associates (SGNA), to stay up-to-date with emerging practices and advancements in the field.

5. Networking and professional involvement: Engage with professional organizations to connect with other gastroenterology nurses, access educational resources, and stay informed about career opportunities. Participate in conferences, webinars, or local chapter meetings to expand your knowledge and network with professionals in the field.

Remember that specific requirements and preferences may vary depending on the healthcare organization, geographical location, and level of experience desired for gastroenterology nursing positions.

| Ostomy Nursing |

Ostomy nursing is a specialized field that focuses on the care of individuals with ostomies, which are surgically created openings on the body for the elimination of bodily waste. Ostomy nurses work in various healthcare settings, including hospitals, home care agencies, and outpatient clinics. They play a crucial role in providing education, support, and direct care to individuals with ostomies. Ostomy nurses help patients adapt to living with an ostomy, manage ostomy appliances, prevent complications, and promote overall well-being.

A Day in the Life

A typical day in the life of an ostomy nurse may involve:

1. Assessing patients with ostomies, including evaluating the stoma, peristomal skin, and overall health status.

2. Assisting patients in the selection, application, and care of ostomy appliances, such as pouching systems and accessories.

3. Educating patients and their families on ostomy care, including proper hygiene, appliance changes, diet modifications, and addressing psychosocial concerns.

4. Managing complications associated with ostomies, such as skin irritation, leakage, peristomal infections, or blockages.

5. Collaborating with other healthcare professionals, including surgeons, wound care specialists, and enterostomal therapists, to develop and implement comprehensive care plans.

6. Providing emotional support and counseling to patients, addressing body image concerns, coping strategies, and promoting self-esteem.

7. Monitoring and managing post-operative recovery and wound healing, ensuring proper stoma function and patient comfort.

8. Facilitating patient and caregiver support groups, workshops, or educational sessions on ostomy care and adjustment.

9. Participating in the development of evidence-based practices and protocols for ostomy care.

10. Engaging in ongoing education and professional development to stay updated on the latest advancements in ostomy nursing, new products, and emerging practices.

Degree(s) Required

To become an ostomy nurse, you need to earn a degree in nursing. The two common degree paths are an Associate Degree in Nursing (ADN) or a Bachelor of Science in Nursing (BSN). However, some employers may prefer or require a BSN for ostomy nursing positions due to the

comprehensive knowledge and critical thinking skills gained.

Salary
$66,640 - $110,960

Specialty Certifications Available or Needed
Certification in ostomy nursing can demonstrate specialized knowledge and competence. The Wound, Ostomy and Continence Nursing Certification Board (WOCNCB) offers the Certified Ostomy Nurse (COCN) credential. Eligibility for the COCN certification typically requires a combination of education, clinical experience in ostomy nursing, and successful completion of an exam.

Job Requirements
Ostomy nursing requires a strong foundation in nursing practice, as well as additional knowledge and skills specific to ostomy care. Job requirements may include:

1. Proficiency in assessing and managing patients with ostomies, including knowledge of various types of ostomies (e.g., colostomy, ileostomy, urostomy) and associated care considerations.
2. Understanding of ostomy appliances, including pouching systems, skin barriers, and accessories, and their proper selection, application, and troubleshooting.
3. Familiarity with wound care principles, including wound healing, peristomal skin assessment, prevention, and management of complications.
4. Effective communication and patient education skills to provide comprehensive information to patients and their families about ostomy care, lifestyle modifications, and psychosocial support.
5. Collaboration with the healthcare team, including surgeons, wound care specialists, enterostomal therapists, and social workers, to provide coordinated and patient-centered care.
6. Proficiency in documentation and record-keeping, ensuring accurate and complete documentation of patient assessments, treatment plans, interventions, and responses.
7. Ability to adapt to a dynamic and often emotionally sensitive environment, providing compassionate care to patients adjusting to life with an ostomy.
8. Knowledge of available resources and support organizations for ostomy patients, referring patients to appropriate support groups, community services, or online communities.
9. Ability to provide emotional support, empathy, and counseling to patients and their families during the challenges of living with an ostomy.

10. Ability to stay updated with current research, evidence-based practices, and clinical guidelines related to ostomy nursing.

Miscellaneous Information You Should Know

To enter the ostomy nursing specialty, you may consider the following:

1. Gain clinical experience in wound care or related areas: Acquire experience in wound care clinics, home health agencies, or surgical units to develop a foundation in managing patients with wounds, understanding wound healing principles, and assisting in ostomy care.

2. Pursue additional education or certifications in ostomy nursing: Consider attending workshops, seminars, or specialized training programs in ostomy nursing to enhance your knowledge and skills. These programs can provide education on ostomy assessment, appliance management, patient education, and evidence-based practices in ostomy care.

3. Stay updated with evidence-based practices: Keep yourself informed about current research, evidence-based practices, and clinical guidelines related to ostomy nursing. Access resources provided by professional organizations, such as the Wound, Ostomy and Continence Nurses Society (WOCN), to stay up-to-date with emerging practices and advancements in the field.

4. Networking and professional involvement: Engage with professional organizations and communities focused on ostomy nursing to connect with other ostomy nurses, access educational resources, and stay informed about career opportunities. Participate in conferences, webinars, or local chapter meetings to expand your knowledge and network with professionals in the field.

Remember that specific requirements and preferences may vary depending on the healthcare organization, geographical location, and level of experience desired for ostomy nursing positions.

| Infusion Nursing |

Infusion nursing is a specialized field that focuses on the administration of medications, fluids, blood products, or other therapies via intravenous (IV) routes. Infusion nurses work in various healthcare settings, including hospitals, clinics, infusion centers, or home healthcare agencies. They play a critical role in assessing patients' needs, ensuring proper infusion technique and safety, monitoring patients' responses to treatments, and providing education and support to patients and their families.

A Day in the Life
A typical day in the life of an infusion nurse may involve:

1. Reviewing patients' medical histories, assessing their vascular access needs, and planning infusion therapy based on prescribed treatments or orders.
2. Initiating and maintaining peripheral or central venous access devices, such as IV catheters, peripherally inserted central catheters (PICCs), or implanted ports.
3. Preparing and administering medications, fluids, blood products, or other intravenous therapies following proper aseptic techniques and safety guidelines.
4. Monitoring patients' vital signs, infusion rates, and overall well-being during infusion therapy to ensure proper administration and identify potential complications.
5. Assessing and managing infusion-related complications, such as infiltration, phlebitis, or catheter-related infections.
6. Educating patients and their families on infusion therapy, including the purpose of treatments, potential side effects, self-care techniques, and signs of complications.
7. Collaborating with the healthcare team, including physicians, pharmacists, and other healthcare professionals, to coordinate care, ensure proper medication orders, and monitor patients' responses to therapy.
8. Documenting patient assessments, interventions, and responses accurately and maintaining proper records.
9. Engaging in ongoing education and professional development to stay updated on the latest advancements in infusion nursing, vascular access devices, and infusion-related technologies.
10. Collaborating with equipment vendors and participating in quality improvement initiatives to enhance infusion practices and patient safety.

Degree(s) Required
To become an infusion nurse, you need to earn a degree in nursing. The

two common degree paths are an Associate Degree in Nursing (ADN) or a Bachelor of Science in Nursing (BSN). However, some employers may prefer or require a BSN for infusion nursing positions due to the comprehensive knowledge and critical thinking skills gained.

Salary
$66,640 - $110,930

Specialty Certifications Available or Needed
Certification in infusion nursing can demonstrate specialized knowledge and competence. The Infusion Nurses Certification Corporation (INCC) offers the Certified Registered Nurse Infusion (CRNI) credential. Eligibility for the CRNI certification typically requires a combination of education, clinical experience, and the successful completion of an exam.

Job Requirements
Infusion nursing requires a strong foundation in medical-surgical nursing skills, as well as additional knowledge and skills specific to intravenous therapy and vascular access. Job requirements may include:

1. Proficiency in assessing and selecting appropriate vascular access devices based on patients' needs, treatment requirements, and duration of therapy.
2. Knowledge of infusion-related procedures, such as medication calculations, IV push administration, blood transfusions, or specialized infusions, following established protocols and guidelines.
3. Competence in administering medications and fluids via various IV routes, including peripheral, central, or peripherally inserted central catheters.
4. Skill in assessing and managing potential complications related to infusion therapy, such as infiltration, extravasation, infection, or catheter-related bloodstream infections.
5. Understanding of sterile techniques, aseptic practices, and infection prevention measures to minimize the risk of infections associated with infusion therapy.
6. Effective communication skills to educate patients and their families on infusion therapy, promote self-care techniques, and address their concerns and questions.
7. Collaboration with the healthcare team, including physicians, pharmacists, and other healthcare professionals, to ensure accurate medication orders, address medication interactions, and monitor patients' responses to therapy.
8. Proficiency in documentation and record-keeping, ensuring accurate

and complete documentation of infusion therapy, including medication administration, patient assessments, and catheter care.

Miscellaneous Information You Should Know

To enter the infusion nursing specialty, you may consider the following:

1. Gain clinical experience in relevant areas: Acquire experience in medical-surgical units, critical care settings, or IV therapy teams to develop a foundation in intravenous therapy, vascular access, and managing infusion-related complications.

2. Pursue additional education or certifications in infusion nursing: Consider attending workshops, seminars, or specialized training programs in infusion nursing to enhance your knowledge and skills. These programs can provide additional education on IV therapy techniques, specialized infusions, vascular access device selection, and complications management.

3. Develop effective communication and patient education skills: Effective communication is crucial in infusion nursing to provide education, support, and guidance to patients and their families. Enhance your ability to communicate complex information in a clear and empathetic manner, adapting your communication style to patients' and families' needs and cultural backgrounds.

4. Stay updated with evidence-based practices: Keep yourself informed about current research, evidence-based practices, and clinical guidelines related to infusion nursing, vascular access, and infection prevention. Access resources provided by professional organizations, such as the Infusion Nurses Society (INS), to stay up-to-date with emerging practices and advancements in the field.

5. Networking and professional involvement: Engage with professional organizations to connect with other infusion nurses, access educational resources, and stay informed about career opportunities. Participate in conferences, webinars, or local chapter meetings to expand your knowledge and network with professionals in the field.

Remember that specific requirements and preferences may vary depending on the healthcare organization, geographical location, and level of experience desired for infusion nursing positions.

| Palliative Care Nursing |

Palliative care nursing is a specialized field that focuses on providing holistic care to patients with serious illnesses and their families. Palliative care nurses aim to enhance the quality of life for patients by addressing their physical, emotional, social, and spiritual needs. They work collaboratively with interdisciplinary teams to provide symptom management, pain relief, and support to patients and their families throughout the continuum of care, from diagnosis to end-of-life.

A Day in the Life

A typical day in the life of a palliative care nurse may involve:

1. Assessing and managing physical symptoms, such as pain, nausea, fatigue, dyspnea, or other distressing symptoms, through appropriate interventions and medications.

2. Providing emotional support and counseling to patients and their families, addressing fears, anxiety, grief, and facilitating open communication.

3. Collaborating with the interdisciplinary team, including physicians, social workers, chaplains, and other healthcare professionals, to develop and implement individualized care plans.

4. Educating patients and their families about the disease process, treatment options, and the goals and benefits of palliative care.

5. Assisting in advance care planning, including discussions about end-of-life care preferences, goals, and the development of care directives.

6. Facilitating effective communication between patients, families, and healthcare providers to ensure that patients' wishes and goals are respected.

7. Coordinating and providing care in various healthcare settings, such as hospitals, hospices, home care, or long-term care facilities.

8. Managing complex ethical and psychosocial issues that arise in palliative care, ensuring patients' dignity, autonomy, and cultural preferences.

9. Providing support to the family caregivers, offering respite care, education, and assistance with the emotional and physical demands of caregiving.

10. Engaging in ongoing education and professional development to stay updated on the latest advancements in palliative care, pain management, and psychosocial support.

Degree(s) Required

To become a palliative care nurse, you need to earn a degree in nursing. The two common degree paths are an Associate Degree in Nursing (ADN) or a Bachelor of Science in Nursing (BSN). However, some employers may prefer or require a BSN for palliative care nursing positions due to the comprehensive knowledge and critical thinking skills gained.

Salary
$66,640 - $110,930

Specialty Certifications Available or Needed
Certification in palliative care nursing can demonstrate specialized knowledge and competence. The Hospice and Palliative Credentialing Center (HPCC) offers the Advanced Certified Hospice and Palliative Nurse (ACHPN) credential. Eligibility for the ACHPN certification typically requires a combination of education, clinical experience in palliative care nursing, and successful completion of an exam.

Job Requirements
Palliative care nursing requires a strong foundation in nursing practice, as well as additional knowledge and skills specific to palliative care. Job requirements may include:

1. Proficiency in assessing and managing physical symptoms, such as pain, dyspnea, nausea, or other distressing symptoms, using evidence-based interventions and pharmacological and non-pharmacological approaches.

2. Understanding of the principles of pain and symptom management, including the use of opioids, adjuvant medications, and non-pharmacological therapies.

3. Familiarity with the psychosocial and emotional aspects of serious illness and end-of-life care, including grief and loss, family dynamics, and cultural considerations.

4. Effective communication and counseling skills to provide compassionate support to patients and families, facilitating discussions about prognosis, goals of care, and advance care planning.

5. Collaboration with the interdisciplinary team, including physicians, social workers, chaplains, and other healthcare professionals, to provide comprehensive care and support to patients and families.

6. Proficiency in documentation and record-keeping, ensuring accurate and thorough documentation of assessments, care plans, interventions, and patient responses.

7. Ability to navigate ethical and legal considerations in palliative care, respecting patients' autonomy, privacy, and confidentiality.

8. Knowledge of available community resources, support groups, and services for patients and families in need of additional support during the palliative care journey.

9. Ability to provide emotional support, empathy, and counseling to patients and families facing serious illness and end-of-life decisions.

10. Ability to stay updated with current research, evidence-based practices, and clinical guidelines related to palliative care.

Miscellaneous Information You Should Know

To enter the palliative care nursing specialty, you may consider the following:

1. Gain clinical experience in hospice or palliative care: Acquire experience in settings that specialize in hospice or palliative care, such as hospices, hospitals with palliative care programs, or home care agencies, to develop a foundation in providing holistic care to patients with serious illnesses.

2. Pursue additional education or certifications in palliative care nursing: Consider attending workshops, seminars, or specialized training programs in palliative care nursing to enhance your knowledge and skills. These programs can provide education on pain and symptom management, communication techniques, ethical considerations, and the provision of psychosocial support in palliative care.

3. Stay updated with evidence-based practices: Keep yourself informed about current research, evidence-based practices, and clinical guidelines related to palliative care. Access resources provided by professional organizations, such as the Hospice and Palliative Nurses Association (HPNA), to stay up-to-date with emerging practices and advancements in the field.

4. Networking and professional involvement: Engage with professional organizations and communities focused on palliative care nursing to connect with other palliative care nurses, access educational resources, and stay informed about career opportunities. Participate in conferences, webinars, or local chapter meetings to expand your knowledge and network with professionals in the field.

Remember that specific requirements and preferences may vary depending on the healthcare organization, geographical location, and level of experience desired for palliative care nursing positions.

| Perianesthesia Nursing |

Perianesthesia nursing, also known as post-anesthesia care unit (PACU) nursing, is a specialized field that focuses on the care of patients before and after anesthesia. Perianesthesia nurses play a crucial role in monitoring patients' vital signs, managing pain and discomfort, assessing for complications, and ensuring a smooth recovery from anesthesia. They work in various settings, including hospitals, surgical centers, and outpatient clinics, collaborating with the anesthesia team and other healthcare professionals to provide safe and effective care.

A Day in the Life
A typical day in the life of a perianesthesia nurse may involve:

1. Assessing patients' preoperative status, reviewing medical histories, and verifying the completion of necessary preoperative procedures.
2. Collaborating with the anesthesia team to ensure proper patient positioning, administering anesthesia, and monitoring patients' responses during surgery.
3. Managing patients' pain and discomfort following surgery, administering medications, and utilizing non-pharmacological interventions to provide comfort.
4. Monitoring vital signs, including blood pressure, heart rate, respiratory rate, and oxygen saturation, to detect any signs of complications or instability.
5. Assessing patients for postoperative complications, such as bleeding, infection, respiratory distress, or adverse reactions to anesthesia, and taking appropriate actions.
6. Providing emotional support and education to patients and their families about the recovery process, potential side effects, and self-care measures at home.
7. Collaborating with the surgical team and other healthcare professionals to ensure a smooth transition from the operating room to the PACU and subsequent care units.
8. Documenting patients' assessments, interventions, and responses accurately and promptly, maintaining comprehensive and up-to-date records.
9. Participating in quality improvement initiatives, such as identifying areas for improvement in perianesthesia care and implementing evidence-based practices.
10. Engaging in ongoing education and professional development to stay updated on the latest advancements in perianesthesia nursing, anesthesia techniques, and patient safety.

Degree(s) Required

To become a perianesthesia nurse, you need to earn a degree in nursing. The two common degree paths are an Associate Degree in Nursing (ADN) or a Bachelor of Science in Nursing (BSN). However, some employers may prefer or require a BSN for perianesthesia nursing positions due to the comprehensive knowledge and critical thinking skills gained.

Salary

$66,640 - $110,930

Specialty Certifications Available or Needed

Certification in perianesthesia nursing can demonstrate specialized knowledge and competence. The American Board of Perianesthesia Nursing Certification (ABPANC) offers the Certified Post Anesthesia Nurse (CPAN) and Certified Ambulatory Perianesthesia Nurse (CAPA) credentials. Eligibility for these certifications typically requires a combination of education, clinical experience in perianesthesia nursing, and successful completion of an exam.

Job Requirements

Perianesthesia nursing requires a strong foundation in nursing practice, as well as additional knowledge and skills specific to perianesthesia care. Job requirements may include:

1. Proficiency in assessing and monitoring patients' vital signs, including blood pressure, heart rate, respiratory rate, oxygen saturation, and pain levels.
2. Understanding of anesthesia techniques, medications, and potential complications, such as allergic reactions, airway obstruction, or malignant hyperthermia.
3. Familiarity with common surgical procedures and their associated postoperative care needs.
4. Effective communication and patient education skills to provide comprehensive information to patients and their families about the recovery process, potential side effects, and self-care measures.
5. Collaboration with the anesthesia team, surgeons, and other healthcare professionals to ensure coordinated and safe care for patients throughout the perianesthesia period.
6. Proficiency in documentation and record-keeping, ensuring accurate and thorough documentation of assessments, interventions, and patient responses.
7. Ability to prioritize and respond quickly to changes in patients'

conditions, identifying and managing emergent situations.

8. Knowledge of pain management techniques and the administration of analgesics and other medications commonly used in the perianesthesia setting.

9. Ability to provide emotional support, empathy, and counseling to patients and their families during the postoperative period.

10. Ability to stay updated with current research, evidence-based practices, and clinical guidelines related to perianesthesia nursing.

Miscellaneous Information You Should Know

To enter the perianesthesia nursing specialty, you may consider the following:

1. Gain clinical experience in perioperative or critical care settings: Acquire experience in areas such as operating rooms, surgical units, or intensive care units to develop a foundation in caring for patients before and after anesthesia administration.

2. Pursue additional education or certifications in perianesthesia nursing: Consider attending workshops, seminars, or specialized training programs in perianesthesia nursing to enhance your knowledge and skills. These programs can provide education on perianesthesia assessments, pain management, anesthesia techniques, and evidence-based practices in perianesthesia care.

3. Stay updated with evidence-based practices: Keep yourself informed about current research, evidence-based practices, and clinical guidelines related to perianesthesia nursing. Access resources provided by professional organizations, such as the American Society of PeriAnesthesia Nurses (ASPAN), to stay up-to-date with emerging practices and advancements in the field.

4. Networking and professional involvement: Engage with professional organizations and communities focused on perianesthesia nursing to connect with other perianesthesia nurses, access educational resources, and stay informed about career opportunities. Participate in conferences, webinars, or local chapter meetings to expand your knowledge and network with professionals in the field.

Remember that specific requirements and preferences may vary depending on the healthcare organization, geographical location, and level of experience desired for perianesthesia nursing positions.

| Vascular Nursing |

Vascular Nursing is a specialized field of nursing that focuses on the care and treatment of patients with vascular conditions, disorders, and diseases. Vascular Nurses work closely with patients who have conditions affecting the arteries, veins, and lymphatic system. They provide care and support throughout the patient's vascular health journey, from prevention and diagnosis to treatment and recovery. Vascular Nurses play a crucial role in managing vascular conditions such as peripheral artery disease, deep vein thrombosis, varicose veins, and arterial aneurysms.

A Day in the Life
A typical day in the life of a Vascular Nurse may involve:

1. Patient Assessment: Conducting comprehensive assessments of patients with vascular conditions, including obtaining medical histories, performing physical examinations, and assessing symptoms related to circulatory problems.

2. Diagnostic Procedures: Assisting with or performing diagnostic tests and procedures such as vascular ultrasounds, angiograms, and Doppler studies to evaluate blood flow and detect vascular abnormalities.

3. Medication Administration: Administering medications as prescribed, including anticoagulants, vasodilators, and antibiotics, and monitoring patients for potential side effects or complications.

4. Wound Care: Providing wound care for patients with vascular ulcers or post-operative incisions. This may involve dressing changes, assessing wound healing progress, and providing patient education on self-care.

5. Surgical Assistance: Assisting vascular surgeons during surgical procedures, such as endovascular interventions, bypass grafting, or vein stripping. Preparing patients for surgery, ensuring proper positioning, and providing post-operative care and monitoring.

6. Patient Education: Educating patients and their families about vascular conditions, treatment options, and self-management strategies. This includes teaching about lifestyle modifications, medication adherence, and signs and symptoms of complications.

7. Vascular Access Management: Monitoring and managing vascular access devices, such as central venous catheters, arterial lines, or peripherally inserted central catheters (PICCs). This includes proper insertion, maintenance, and preventing complications like infection or thrombosis.

8. Collaborative Care: Collaborating with vascular surgeons, interventional radiologists, wound care specialists, and other healthcare professionals to develop and implement individualized care plans for

patients. This includes ongoing communication and coordination of care to ensure optimal patient outcomes.

9. Patient Support: Providing emotional support and counseling to patients and their families as they navigate their vascular conditions and treatments. Assisting with coping strategies, addressing concerns, and facilitating access to additional resources.

10. Documentation: Ensuring accurate and thorough documentation of patient assessments, interventions, and outcomes in medical records. Adhering to legal and ethical standards for documentation and maintaining patient privacy and confidentiality.

Degree(s) Required

To become a Vascular Nurse, you need to earn a degree in nursing. The two common degree paths are an Associate Degree in Nursing (ADN) or a Bachelor of Science in Nursing (BSN). However, some employers may prefer or require a BSN due to its comprehensive curriculum and broader range of nursing skills.

Salary
$68,450 - $115,800

Specialty Certifications Available or Needed

Obtaining specialty certification in Vascular Nursing can validate advanced knowledge and expertise in this field. The Vascular Nursing Certification offered by the Society for Vascular Nursing (SVN) is available for nurses who meet the eligibility criteria and successfully pass the certification exam. This certification demonstrates specialized knowledge in vascular nursing and signifies a commitment to professional growth and excellence.

Job Requirements

Vascular Nurses require specific knowledge and skills to provide effective care to patients with vascular conditions. Job requirements may include:

1. Vascular Knowledge: Acquire a solid understanding of vascular anatomy, physiology, and common vascular conditions such as peripheral artery disease, venous insufficiency, arterial aneurysms, and deep vein thrombosis.

2. Diagnostic and Interventional Procedures: Familiarity with diagnostic procedures such as Doppler ultrasounds, angiography, and venous studies. Knowledge of interventional procedures like angioplasty, stenting, or thrombectomy performed by vascular surgeons or interventional

radiologists.

3. Medication Management: Proficiency in administering and managing medications commonly used in vascular care, including anticoagulants, antiplatelet agents, vasodilators, and thrombolytics.

4. Wound Care: Competence in managing vascular ulcers, including wound assessment, dressing selection, infection prevention, and implementing strategies to promote wound healing.

5. Surgical Assistance: Assisting with vascular surgeries, including pre-operative and post-operative care, instrument preparation, and patient monitoring during procedures.

6. Patient Education: Ability to effectively educate patients and their families about vascular conditions, treatment options, lifestyle modifications, and self-care measures to promote vascular health and prevent complications.

7. Collaboration and Communication: Collaborating with vascular surgeons, interventional radiologists, wound care specialists, and other healthcare professionals to provide comprehensive and coordinated care. Effective communication and interdisciplinary teamwork are essential.

8. Vascular Access Management: Competence in managing and maintaining various vascular access devices, such as central venous catheters, arterial lines, or PICCs. This includes proper insertion techniques, monitoring for complications, and implementing infection prevention strategies.

9. Documentation: Ensuring accurate and thorough documentation of patient assessments, interventions, and outcomes in medical records. Adhering to legal and ethical standards for documentation.

10. Continual Learning: Staying updated on current research, evidence-based practices, and advancements in vascular care through professional development activities, attending conferences, and participating in vascular-specific workshops and seminars.

Miscellaneous Information You Should Know

To enter the Vascular Nursing specialty, you may consider the following:

1. Gain Clinical Experience: Seek opportunities to work in vascular or surgical units during your nursing education or through internships and clinical rotations. This experience will provide exposure to vascular conditions, diagnostic procedures, and surgical interventions.

2. Join Professional Organizations: Consider joining professional organizations, such as the Society for Vascular Nursing (SVN), to access resources, educational opportunities, and networking events specific to vascular nursing.

3. Pursue Continuing Education: Engage in continuing education activities, such as attending vascular conferences, workshops, and webinars, to stay updated on advancements and best practices in vascular care.

4. Seek Mentorship and Collaboration: Connect with experienced Vascular Nurses, vascular surgeons, or interventional radiologists who can serve as mentors and provide guidance as you develop your vascular nursing skills.

5. Specialty Training Programs: Explore specialized training programs or fellowships in vascular nursing offered by healthcare institutions or professional organizations to enhance your

knowledge and skills in this field.

Remember that specific requirements and preferences may vary depending on the employer, healthcare facility, or vascular practice where you plan to practice as a Vascular Nurse.

| Rehabilitation Nursing |

Rehabilitation nursing, also known as rehab nursing, is a specialized field that focuses on providing care to individuals with disabilities or chronic illnesses to help them regain or improve their physical, cognitive, and emotional functioning. Rehabilitation nurses work in various settings, including hospitals, rehabilitation centers, long-term care facilities, and home care. They collaborate with interdisciplinary teams to develop and implement personalized care plans, facilitate rehabilitation therapies, and support patients in achieving their maximum level of independence and quality of life.

A Day in the Life

A typical day in the life of a rehabilitation nurse may involve:

1. Patient Assessment and Care Planning: Conducting comprehensive assessments of patients' physical, cognitive, and psychosocial status to develop individualized care plans. Collaborating with the interdisciplinary team, including physical therapists, occupational therapists, speech therapists, and social workers, to establish goals and interventions.

2. Rehabilitation Therapy Assistance: Assisting patients with therapeutic activities, mobility exercises, and rehabilitative techniques to improve strength, endurance, coordination, and independence.

3. Medication Administration and Management: Administering medications as prescribed and monitoring their effectiveness and potential side effects. Educating patients and their families about medication regimens, including proper administration and potential interactions.

4. Wound Care and Management: Providing wound care, including dressing changes, wound assessments, and monitoring for signs of infection. Collaborating with wound care specialists when necessary.

5. Patient and Family Education: Educating patients and their families about their conditions, rehabilitation goals, and strategies to optimize recovery and self-care. Providing guidance on adaptive techniques and equipment to enhance independence.

6. Emotional Support: Providing emotional support to patients and their families, addressing psychological and social challenges associated with disabilities or chronic illnesses. Collaborating with psychologists or counselors to facilitate psychological adjustment and coping.

7. Collaborative Care: Collaborating with physical therapists, occupational therapists, and speech therapists to coordinate rehabilitation interventions and monitor progress towards goals. Communicating regularly with the interdisciplinary team to ensure cohesive and comprehensive care.

8. Discharge Planning and Transition: Participating in discharge

planning and coordinating resources for patients' transition from the rehabilitation setting to home or another care setting. Providing education on post-discharge care, community resources, and follow-up appointments.

9. Documentation and Record-Keeping: Maintaining accurate and detailed documentation of patient assessments, care plans, interventions, progress notes, and discharge summaries. Ensuring compliance with regulatory standards and healthcare policies.

10. Ongoing Education: Engaging in continuous learning and professional development to stay updated on evidence-based practices in rehabilitation nursing. Participating in training programs, workshops, and conferences to enhance knowledge and skills in rehabilitation nursing.

Degree(s) Required

To become a rehabilitation nurse, you need to earn a degree in nursing. The two common degree paths are an Associate Degree in Nursing (ADN) or a Bachelor of Science in Nursing (BSN). However, some employers may prefer or require a BSN for rehabilitation nursing positions due to the comprehensive knowledge and critical thinking skills gained.

Salary

$66,640 - $110,930

Specialty Certifications Available or Needed

Certification in rehabilitation nursing can demonstrate specialized knowledge and competence. The Rehabilitation Nursing Certification Board (RNCB) offers the Certified Rehabilitation Registered Nurse (CRRN) credential. Eligibility for the CRRN certification typically requires a combination of education, clinical experience in rehabilitation nursing, and successful completion of an exam.

Job Requirements

Rehabilitation nursing requires a strong foundation in nursing practice, as well as additional knowledge and skills specific to rehabilitation care. Job requirements may include:

1. Knowledge of physical and cognitive rehabilitation techniques, including mobility exercises, therapeutic activities, and adaptive equipment.
2. Understanding of common disabilities and chronic illnesses requiring rehabilitation, such as stroke, spinal cord injuries, traumatic brain injuries, amputations, and orthopedic conditions.
3. Proficiency in patient assessment and care planning, including functional assessments, neurological assessments, and identification of rehabilitation goals.

4. Familiarity with rehabilitation therapies, including physical therapy, occupational therapy, speech therapy, and recreational therapy, to collaborate effectively with the interdisciplinary team.

5. Competence in wound care management, including assessment, dressing changes, and prevention of complications.

6. Ability to provide patient and family education on rehabilitation goals, strategies, and community resources to support optimal recovery and self-management.

7. Collaboration and communication skills to work effectively with interdisciplinary teams, patients, families, and community resources.

8. Ability to provide emotional support, empathy, and counseling to patients and families facing the challenges of disabilities or chronic illnesses.

9. Documentation and record-keeping skills to maintain accurate and detailed patient records, including assessments, care plans, interventions, progress notes, and discharge summaries.

10. Ability to stay updated with current research, evidence-based practices, and clinical guidelines related to rehabilitation nursing.

Miscellaneous Information You Should Know

To enter the rehabilitation nursing specialty, you may consider the following:

1. Gain clinical experience in rehabilitation settings: Seek opportunities to gain experience in rehabilitation units, long-term care facilities, or home care settings. This experience will provide valuable exposure to rehabilitation care, interdisciplinary teamwork, and patient-centered approaches.

2. Pursue additional education or certifications in rehabilitation nursing: Consider attending workshops, seminars, or specialized training programs in rehabilitation nursing to enhance your knowledge and skills. These programs can provide education on rehabilitation techniques, patient assessment, adaptive equipment, and evidence-based practices in rehabilitation nursing.

3. Stay informed about current research, evidence-based practices, and clinical guidelines related to rehabilitation nursing. Access resources provided by professional organizations, such as the Association of Rehabilitation Nurses (ARN).

4. Networking and professional involvement: Engage with professional organizations and communities focused on rehabilitation nursing to connect with other rehabilitation nurses, access educational resources, and stay informed about career opportunities.

Remember that specific requirements and preferences may vary depending on the healthcare organization, geographical location, and experience level desired for rehabilitation nursing positions.

| Flight Nursing |

Flight nursing involves providing critical care and emergency medical services to patients during air transport, such as helicopter or fixed-wing aircraft. Flight nurses work in aeromedical transport teams and are responsible for providing high-quality patient care in challenging and dynamic environments. They stabilize and manage patients with complex medical conditions or trauma during transport, often in remote or austere locations. Flight nursing requires advanced clinical skills, critical thinking, and the ability to make rapid decisions in high-pressure situations.

A Day in the Life
A typical day in the life of a flight nurse may involve:

1. Receiving a patient transfer request from a referring facility or emergency response team.
2. Conducting a thorough assessment of the patient's condition and preparing for air transport, considering factors like weather conditions and flight safety.
3. Collaborating with the flight crew, such as pilots and paramedics, to ensure a smooth and safe transport process.
4. Administering advanced life support interventions, such as medication administration, cardiac monitoring, or airway management, as necessary.
5. Providing ongoing monitoring and critical care interventions during the transport, adapting to the changing needs and conditions of the patient.
6. Communicating with the receiving facility or medical control to provide updates on the patient's condition and coordinate appropriate care upon arrival.
7. Collaborating with the healthcare team to ensure continuity of care and seamless transitions for the patient.
8. Documenting patient assessments, interventions, and any pertinent information accurately and efficiently.
9. Participating in continuing education and skills training to maintain proficiency in flight nursing and keep up-to-date with advancements in aeromedical transport.

Degree(s) Required
To become a flight nurse, you need to earn a degree in nursing. The two common degree paths are an Associate Degree in Nursing (ADN) or a Bachelor of Science in Nursing (BSN). However, many employers prefer or require a BSN for flight nursing positions due to the advanced clinical skills and critical thinking required for this specialty. Additionally, obtaining

advanced certifications or specialized training in critical care can enhance your knowledge and skills in this field.

Salary
$68,910 - $112,210

Specialty Certifications Available or Needed
Certification in critical care or flight nursing can demonstrate specialized knowledge and competence as a flight nurse. The Board of Certification for Emergency Nursing (BCEN) offers the Certified Flight Registered Nurse (CFRN) credential. Eligibility for the CFRN certification typically requires a combination of education, clinical experience, and the successful completion of an exam.

Job Requirements
Flight nursing requires exceptional clinical skills, critical thinking abilities, and the ability to work effectively in high-stress environments. Job requirements may include:

1. Proficiency in advanced life support interventions and critical care skills, such as cardiac monitoring, medication administration, and advanced airway management.

2. Knowledge of critical care principles, trauma management, and emergency medical practices.

3. Competence in assessing and managing patients with complex medical conditions, including trauma, cardiac emergencies, or acute respiratory distress.

4. Ability to make rapid decisions and adapt to changing patient conditions during the transport process.

5. Effective communication and collaboration skills to work closely with the flight crew, referring facilities, and receiving hospitals.

6. Understanding of flight safety protocols and adherence to standard operating procedures.

7. Skill in working with specialized equipment used in aeromedical transport, such as ventilators, defibrillators, or transport monitors.

8. Proficiency in documentation and record-keeping, ensuring accurate and complete documentation of patient encounters.

Miscellaneous Information You Should Know
To enter the flight nursing specialty, you may consider the following:

1. Acquire relevant clinical experience: Gain experience in critical care settings, such as intensive care units (ICUs), emergency departments (EDs),

or trauma centers. This experience will provide a foundation in managing critically ill or injured patients and developing clinical skills necessary for flight nursing.

2. Obtain certifications in critical care and advanced life support: Consider obtaining certifications such as the Critical Care Registered Nurse (CCRN) credential or advanced life support certifications like Advanced Cardiac Life Support (ACLS) and Pediatric Advanced Life Support (PALS). These certifications demonstrate your advanced knowledge and competence in critical care and emergency interventions.

3. Pursue additional training in flight nursing: Seek out educational programs or specialized training courses that focus on flight nursing. These programs may cover topics such as aeromedical transport, aviation safety, and managing patients in challenging environments.

4. Develop strong communication and teamwork skills: Effective communication and teamwork are vital in flight nursing, as you will work closely with the flight crew, paramedics, and receiving healthcare teams. Enhance your communication skills to ensure clear and concise information exchange during critical moments.

5. Meet physical requirements: Flight nursing may involve physical demands such as lifting, carrying, and maneuvering patients in confined spaces. Ensure you meet the physical requirements set by your employer or aeromedical transport company.

6. Maintain flexibility and adaptability: Flight nursing often requires working in unpredictable environments and responding to emergent situations. Develop the ability to adapt to changing circumstances and remain calm under pressure.

Remember that specific requirements and preferences may vary depending on the healthcare organization, geographical location, and level of experience desired for flight nursing positions. Additionally, aeromedical transport companies may have specific requirements for flight nurses, such as flight experience or additional certifications beyond those mentioned here.

| Hospice Nursing |

Hospice nursing is a specialized field that focuses on providing compassionate care to patients with terminal illnesses and their families. Hospice nurses work in hospice centers, hospitals, long-term care facilities, or patients' homes. They focus on managing pain and symptoms, providing emotional support, facilitating end-of-life discussions, and ensuring a comfortable and dignified transition for patients and their families.

A Day in the Life

A typical day in the life of a hospice nurse may involve:

1. Collaborating with the interdisciplinary hospice team to assess patients' physical, emotional, and spiritual needs.

2. Providing comprehensive nursing assessments, including pain and symptom management, and developing individualized care plans.

3. Administering medications, including pain medications and comfort measures, and managing patients' symptoms to enhance their quality of life.

4. Educating patients and families about the disease process, treatment options, pain management techniques, and end-of-life care decisions.

5. Assisting patients and families in creating advance care plans, including discussing and documenting their preferences for care and resuscitation.

6. Offering emotional support and counseling to patients and their families, providing a listening ear, addressing their concerns, and facilitating end-of-life discussions.

7. Coordinating and collaborating with the interdisciplinary team, including physicians, social workers, chaplains, and bereavement counselors, to provide comprehensive care.

8. Conducting regular visits to patients' homes or care facilities to assess their needs, monitor their condition, and ensure effective symptom management.

9. Documenting patient assessments, interventions, and responses accurately and maintaining proper records.

10. Engaging in self-care practices and seeking support from colleagues and supervisors to manage the emotional and psychological demands of hospice nursing.

Degree(s) Required

To become a hospice nurse, you need to earn a degree in nursing. The two common degree paths are an Associate Degree in Nursing (ADN) or a Bachelor of Science in Nursing (BSN). However, some employers may prefer or require a BSN for hospice nursing positions due to the

comprehensive knowledge and critical thinking skills gained.

Salary
$66,640 - $110,930

Specialty Certifications Available or Needed
Certification in hospice and palliative nursing can demonstrate specialized knowledge and competence. The Hospice and Palliative Credentialing Center (HPCC) offers the Certified Hospice and Palliative Nurse (CHPN) credential. Eligibility for the CHPN certification typically requires a combination of education, clinical experience, and the successful completion of an exam.

Job Requirements
Hospice nursing requires a strong foundation in medical-surgical nursing skills, as well as additional knowledge and skills specific to providing end-of-life care. Job requirements may include:

1. Proficiency in assessing and managing patients with terminal illnesses, including pain and symptom management, psychosocial support, and coordination of care.
2. Knowledge of hospice philosophy, principles of palliative care, and the physical and emotional aspects of the dying process.
3. Competence in administering medications commonly used in hospice care, including opioids for pain management and other comfort measures.
4. Skill in facilitating discussions about end-of-life care, advance directives, and treatment choices, while respecting patients' autonomy and cultural beliefs.
5. Effective communication skills to provide emotional support, counseling, and education to patients and their families during the end-of-life journey.
6. Understanding of grief and bereavement processes and the ability to provide support to families during and after the loss of a loved one.
7. Collaboration with the interdisciplinary hospice team, including physicians, social workers, chaplains, and bereavement counselors, to provide holistic care.
8. Proficiency in documentation and record-keeping, ensuring accurate and complete documentation of patient assessments, care plans, and interventions.

Miscellaneous Information You Should Know
To enter the hospice nursing specialty, you may consider the following:

1. Gain clinical experience in relevant areas: Acquire experience in medical-surgical units, oncology units, or palliative care settings to develop a foundation in managing patients with serious illnesses and end-of-life care.

2. Develop effective communication and counseling skills: Effective communication is crucial in hospice nursing to establish trust, provide emotional support, and facilitate end-of-life discussions. Enhance your ability to communicate sensitively and empathetically with patients and families, actively listen, and address their concerns.

3. Participate in training or educational programs in hospice and palliative care: Seek opportunities to attend workshops, seminars, or specialized training programs focused on hospice and palliative care. These programs can provide additional education on pain and symptom management, psychosocial support, and grief counseling.

4. Build resilience and self-care strategies: Hospice nursing can be emotionally demanding. Develop strategies to manage stress, enhance self-care practices, and seek support from colleagues, supervisors, or counseling services to maintain your own well-being.

5. Networking and professional involvement: Engage with professional organizations, such as the Hospice and Palliative Nurses Association (HPNA), to connect with other hospice nurses, access educational resources, and stay informed about career opportunities. Participate in conferences, webinars, or local chapter meetings to expand your knowledge and network with professionals in the field.

Remember that specific requirements and preferences may vary depending on the healthcare organization, geographical location, and level of experience desired for hospice nursing positions.

| Pain Management Nursing |

Pain management nursing is a specialized field that focuses on assessing, diagnosing, and managing pain in patients across various healthcare settings. Pain management nurses work closely with patients experiencing acute or chronic pain, helping to alleviate their discomfort and improve their quality of life. They employ a multidimensional approach to pain management, including pharmacological interventions, non-pharmacological techniques, patient education, and support.

A Day in the Life

A typical day in the life of a pain management nurse may involve:

1. Conducting comprehensive pain assessments, including evaluating the intensity, location, quality, and impact of pain on the patient's physical and emotional well-being.

2. Collaborating with the healthcare team to develop individualized pain management plans that consider the patient's medical history, cultural beliefs, and personal preferences.

3. Administering pain medications, such as opioids, non-opioid analgesics, or adjuvant medications, in accordance with prescribed orders and monitoring their effectiveness and side effects.

4. Implementing non-pharmacological pain management interventions, such as relaxation techniques, distraction techniques, therapeutic touch, heat or cold therapy, and positioning strategies.

5. Educating patients and their families about pain management techniques, medication adherence, potential side effects, and the importance of open communication in managing pain.

6. Monitoring and reassessing patients regularly to evaluate the effectiveness of pain management interventions and adjusting the treatment plan as necessary.

7. Collaborating with other healthcare professionals, including physicians, physical therapists, psychologists, and palliative care teams, to provide comprehensive pain management for patients.

8. Providing emotional support and counseling to patients experiencing pain, addressing anxiety, fear, and the psychosocial impact of chronic pain.

9. Advocating for patients' rights to receive adequate pain management, ensuring that pain assessments and interventions are conducted promptly and effectively.

10. Engaging in ongoing education and professional development to stay updated on the latest advancements in pain management, evidence-based practices, and new treatment modalities.

Degree(s) Required

To become a pain management nurse, you need to earn a degree in nursing. The two common degree paths are an Associate Degree in Nursing (ADN) or a Bachelor of Science in Nursing (BSN). However, some employers may prefer or require a BSN for pain management nursing positions due to the comprehensive knowledge and critical thinking skills gained.

Salary

$66,640 - $110,930

Specialty Certifications Available or Needed

Certification in pain management nursing can demonstrate specialized knowledge and competence. The American Society for Pain Management Nursing (ASPMN) offers the Pain Management Nursing Certification (RN-BC) credential. Eligibility for the RN-BC certification typically requires a combination of education, clinical experience in pain management nursing, and successful completion of an exam.

Job Requirements

Pain management nursing requires a strong foundation in nursing practice, as well as additional knowledge and skills specific to pain assessment and management. Job requirements may include:

1. Proficiency in pain assessment techniques, including the use of standardized pain scales, patient self-reporting, and observation of physical and behavioral cues.
2. Understanding of the pharmacology of pain medications, including knowledge of different classes of analgesics, dosage calculations, potential side effects, and drug interactions.
3. Familiarity with non-pharmacological pain management techniques, such as relaxation exercises, guided imagery, cognitive-behavioral therapies, and complementary and alternative therapies.
4. Effective communication and patient education skills to provide comprehensive information to patients and their families about pain management strategies, medication regimens, and self-care techniques.
5. Collaboration with the healthcare team to develop and implement interdisciplinary pain management plans, considering physical, psychological, social, and spiritual aspects of pain.
6. Proficiency in documentation and record-keeping, ensuring accurate and thorough documentation of pain assessments, treatment plans, interventions, and patient responses.
7. Ability to assess and manage both acute and chronic pain conditions,

tailoring interventions to meet individual patient needs and preferences.

8. Knowledge of special populations, such as pediatric or geriatric patients, and the unique considerations involved in pain management for these populations.

9. Ability to provide emotional support, empathy, and counseling to patients and their families dealing with pain and its impact on daily life.

10. Ability to stay updated with current research, evidence-based practices, and clinical guidelines related to pain management.

Miscellaneous Information You Should Know

To enter the pain management nursing specialty, you may consider the following:

1. Gain clinical experience in pain management or related areas: Acquire experience in settings that specialize in pain management, such as pain clinics, palliative care units, or oncology units, to develop a foundation in assessing and managing patients with various types of pain.

2. Pursue additional education or certifications in pain management nursing: Consider attending workshops, seminars, or specialized training programs in pain management nursing to enhance your knowledge and skills. These programs can provide education on pain assessment tools, pharmacological and non-pharmacological interventions, and evidence-based practices in pain management.

3. Stay updated with evidence-based practices: Keep yourself informed about current research, evidence-based practices, and clinical guidelines related to pain management. Access resources provided by professional organizations, such as the American Society for Pain Management Nursing (ASPMN), to stay up-to-date with emerging practices and advancements in the field.

4. Networking and professional involvement: Engage with professional organizations and communities focused on pain management nursing to connect with other pain management nurses, access educational resources, and stay informed about career opportunities. Participate in conferences, webinars, or local chapter meetings to expand your knowledge and network with professionals in the field.

Remember that specific requirements and preferences may vary depending on the healthcare organization, geographical location, and level of experience desired for pain management nursing positions.

| Nuclear Medicine Nursing |

Nuclear medicine nursing is a specialized field that focuses on the use of radioactive materials and nuclear medicine procedures for diagnostic and therapeutic purposes. Nuclear medicine nurses work in healthcare settings such as hospitals, nuclear medicine departments, cancer treatment centers, and research facilities. They play a crucial role in administering radioactive materials, monitoring patient response to treatments, and ensuring safety protocols are followed during nuclear medicine procedures.

A Day in the Life
A typical day in the life of a nuclear medicine nurse may involve:

1. Assessing and preparing patients for nuclear medicine procedures, explaining the procedure, obtaining informed consent, and addressing any concerns or questions.

2. Administering radioactive materials to patients for diagnostic imaging or therapeutic treatments, ensuring proper dosage, following radiation safety protocols, and monitoring patient response.

3. Collaborating with nuclear medicine technologists, radiologists, and other healthcare professionals to plan and coordinate nuclear medicine procedures and treatments.

4. Monitoring patients during nuclear medicine procedures, ensuring patient comfort and safety, and providing emotional support.

5. Collecting and analyzing patient data, including vital signs, laboratory results, and imaging studies, to assess treatment response and identify potential adverse reactions.

6. Educating patients and their families about nuclear medicine procedures, potential side effects, and post-procedure care instructions.

7. Administering medications to manage symptoms or side effects related to nuclear medicine procedures, such as antiemetics or analgesics.

8. Monitoring radiation safety practices and ensuring compliance with regulations and guidelines to protect patients, staff, and the public.

9. Maintaining accurate documentation of patient assessments, treatment procedures, and radiation exposure records.

10. Engaging in ongoing education and professional development to stay updated on the latest advancements in nuclear medicine, radiation safety, and evidence-based practices in nuclear nursing.

Degree(s) Required
To become a nuclear nurse, you need to earn a degree in nursing. The two common degree paths are an Associate Degree in Nursing (ADN) or a Bachelor of Science in Nursing (BSN). However, some employers may

prefer or require a BSN for nuclear nursing positions due to the comprehensive knowledge and critical thinking skills gained.

Salary
$65,000 - $107,500

Specialty Certifications Available or Needed
Certification in nuclear nursing can demonstrate specialized knowledge and competence. The Nuclear Medicine Technology Certification Board (NMTCB) offers the Certified Nuclear Medicine Technologist (CNMT) credential. Although this certification is primarily for technologists, it can be valuable for nuclear nurses who work closely with nuclear medicine technologists and have a strong understanding of nuclear medicine procedures.

Job Requirements
Nuclear nursing requires a strong foundation in nursing practice, as well as additional knowledge and skills specific to nuclear medicine and radiation safety. Job requirements may include:

1. Proficiency in administering and monitoring radioactive materials for diagnostic imaging or therapeutic treatments, including knowledge of radiation physics, radiation safety protocols, and regulations.
2. Understanding of nuclear medicine procedures and their indications, including knowledge of various radioactive tracers, imaging techniques, and therapeutic applications.
3. Knowledge of radiopharmaceuticals, their administration, handling, and potential side effects or adverse reactions.
4. Familiarity with radiation safety practices and regulations to protect patients, staff, and the public from unnecessary radiation exposure.
5. Effective communication skills to provide comprehensive education and support to patients and their families regarding nuclear medicine procedures, radiation safety, and post-procedure care.
6. Collaboration with the healthcare team, including radiologists, nuclear medicine technologists, physicists, and pharmacists, to provide coordinated and patient-centered care.
7. Proficiency in documentation and record-keeping, ensuring accurate and complete documentation of patient assessments, treatment procedures, radiation exposure records, and adherence to safety protocols.
8. Ability to adapt to a dynamic environment, handle emergencies or complications related to nuclear medicine procedures, and make critical decisions to ensure patient safety and well-being.
9. Attention to detail and adherence to strict protocols to minimize

radiation exposure and maintain quality control in nuclear medicine procedures.

10. Continuous monitoring of advancements in nuclear medicine, radiation safety practices, and regulations.

Miscellaneous Information You Should Know

To enter the nuclear nursing specialty, you may consider the following:

1. Gain clinical experience in nuclear medicine or related areas: Acquire experience in nuclear medicine departments, radiology departments, or oncology units to develop a foundation in nuclear medicine procedures, radiation safety practices, and the use of radiopharmaceuticals.

2. Pursue additional education or certifications in nuclear medicine or radiation safety: Consider attending workshops, seminars, or specialized training programs in nuclear medicine or radiation safety to enhance your knowledge and skills. These programs can provide education on radiation safety practices, radiopharmaceuticals, and evidence-based practices in nuclear nursing.

3. Stay updated with evidence-based practices: Keep yourself informed about current research, evidence-based practices, and clinical guidelines related to nuclear nursing. Access resources provided by professional organizations, such as the Society of Nuclear Medicine and Molecular Imaging (SNMMI), to stay up-to-date with emerging practices and advancements in the field.

4. Networking and professional involvement: Engage with professional organizations and communities focused on nuclear nursing or nuclear medicine to connect with other nuclear nurses, access educational resources, and stay informed about career opportunities. Participate in conferences, webinars, or local chapter meetings to expand your knowledge and network with professionals in the field.

Remember that specific requirements and preferences may vary depending on the healthcare organization, geographical location, and level of experience desired for nuclear nursing positions.

| Pulmonary Nursing |

Pulmonary nursing, also known as respiratory nursing, is a specialized field that focuses on providing care to patients with respiratory disorders and conditions, such as asthma, chronic obstructive pulmonary disease (COPD), pneumonia, and cystic fibrosis. Pulmonary nurses play a crucial role in assessing, managing, and educating patients with respiratory problems. They work in various settings, including hospitals, clinics, pulmonary rehabilitation centers, and home care, collaborating with pulmonologists and other healthcare professionals to promote optimal respiratory health.

A Day in the Life

A typical day in the life of a pulmonary nurse may involve:

1. Patient Assessment: Conducting thorough respiratory assessments, including evaluating patients' lung function, respiratory symptoms, oxygen saturation levels, and respiratory distress.

2. Medication Administration: Administering and monitoring the effectiveness of respiratory medications, such as bronchodilators, corticosteroids, and oxygen therapy.

3. Respiratory Interventions: Performing respiratory treatments and interventions, including nebulizer treatments, chest physiotherapy, incentive spirometry, and airway clearance techniques.

4. Monitoring and Evaluation: Monitoring patients' respiratory status, vital signs, and oxygen levels. Assessing and documenting changes in symptoms and lung function.

5. Patient Education: Providing comprehensive education to patients and their families about respiratory disorders, self-management techniques, medication administration, inhaler techniques, and lifestyle modifications.

6. Collaboration with the Healthcare Team: Collaborating with pulmonologists, respiratory therapists, physical therapists, and other healthcare professionals to develop and implement patient care plans.

7. Pulmonary Rehabilitation: Participating in pulmonary rehabilitation programs, assisting patients with exercises, education, and breathing techniques to improve lung function and overall respiratory health.

8. Support for Respiratory Procedures: Assisting with diagnostic procedures, such as pulmonary function tests, bronchoscopy, and arterial blood gas sampling.

9. Patient Advocacy: Advocating for patients' respiratory health needs, ensuring access to appropriate resources, and facilitating coordination of care.

10. Documentation and Record-Keeping: Maintaining accurate and

detailed documentation of patient assessments, interventions, and responses. Ensuring compliance with regulatory standards and healthcare policies.

Degree(s) Required

To become a pulmonary nurse, you need to earn a degree in nursing. The two common degree paths are an Associate Degree in Nursing (ADN) or a Bachelor of Science in Nursing (BSN). However, some employers may prefer or require a BSN for pulmonary nursing positions due to the comprehensive knowledge and critical thinking skills gained.

Salary

$68,450 - $115,800

Specialty Certifications Available or Needed

Certification in pulmonary nursing can demonstrate specialized knowledge and competence. The American Nurses Credentialing Center (ANCC) offers the Pulmonary Care Nursing Certification (PCN-C). Eligibility for the PCN-C certification typically requires a combination of education, clinical experience in pulmonary nursing, and successful completion of an exam.

Job Requirements

Pulmonary nursing requires a strong foundation in nursing practice, as well as additional knowledge and skills specific to respiratory care. Job requirements may include:

1. Proficiency in respiratory assessments, including auscultation, pulse oximetry, spirometry, and arterial blood gas interpretation.
2. Knowledge of respiratory disorders, including asthma, COPD, pneumonia, pulmonary fibrosis, and sleep apnea.
3. Familiarity with respiratory medications, inhalation therapy devices, oxygen therapy, and airway management techniques.
4. Understanding of pulmonary rehabilitation principles and techniques to assist patients in optimizing lung function.
5. Ability to provide patient education on self-management strategies, including medication administration, inhaler techniques, breathing exercises, and lifestyle modifications.
6. Collaboration with the healthcare team to ensure coordinated care, including communication with pulmonologists, respiratory therapists, and other specialists.
7. Proficiency in documentation and record-keeping, ensuring accurate and thorough documentation of assessments, care plans, interventions, and

patient responses.

8. Ability to provide emotional support, empathy, and counseling to patients and families facing respiratory challenges.

9. Knowledge of infection control practices and the ability to implement appropriate precautions in respiratory care.

10. Ability to stay updated with current research, evidence-based practices, and clinical guidelines related to pulmonary nursing.

Miscellaneous Information You Should Know

To enter the pulmonary nursing specialty, you may consider the following:

1. Gain clinical experience in respiratory care: Seek opportunities to gain experience in areas such as respiratory units, pulmonary rehabilitation centers, or critical care settings. This experience will provide valuable exposure to the management of respiratory disorders and interventions.

2. Pursue additional education or certifications in pulmonary nursing: Consider attending workshops, seminars, or specialized training programs in pulmonary nursing to enhance your knowledge and skills. These programs can provide education on respiratory assessments, therapeutic interventions, and evidence-based practices in pulmonary nursing.

3. Stay updated with evidence-based practices: Keep yourself informed about current research, evidence-based practices, and clinical guidelines related to pulmonary nursing. Access resources provided by professional organizations, such as the American Association of Respiratory Care (AARC), to stay up-to-date with emerging practices and advancements in the field.

4. Networking and professional involvement: Engage with professional organizations and communities focused on pulmonary nursing to connect with other pulmonary nurses, access educational resources, and stay informed about career opportunities. Participate in conferences, webinars, or local chapter meetings to expand your knowledge and network with professionals in the field.

Remember that specific requirements and preferences may vary depending on the healthcare organization, geographical location, and level of experience desired for pulmonary nursing positions.

| Long-Term Care Nursing |

Long-term care nursing is a specialized field that focuses on providing care to individuals who require extended assistance due to chronic illnesses, disabilities, or advanced age. Long-term care nurses work in settings such as nursing homes, assisted living facilities, rehabilitation centers, or hospice care. They play a vital role in ensuring the well-being of residents, managing their complex medical needs, promoting quality of life, and providing emotional support to residents and their families.

A Day in the Life

A typical day in the life of a long-term care nurse may involve:

1. Assessing residents' health status, including physical, cognitive, and psychosocial functioning, and developing individualized care plans.

2. Administering medications, treatments, and therapies as prescribed, and managing residents' chronic conditions, such as diabetes, hypertension, or respiratory disorders.

3. Assisting with activities of daily living (ADLs), including bathing, dressing, grooming, and toileting, while promoting residents' independence and dignity.

4. Monitoring residents' vital signs, changes in condition, and response to treatments, promptly reporting any concerns to the healthcare team.

5. Collaborating with interdisciplinary teams, including physicians, therapists, social workers, and dietitians, to provide comprehensive care and address residents' physical, emotional, and social needs.

6. Providing emotional support and companionship to residents, engaging in therapeutic communication, and facilitating social interactions among residents.

7. Educating residents and their families on self-care techniques, managing chronic conditions, medication adherence, and promoting healthy lifestyles.

8. Implementing infection prevention and control measures to maintain a safe and clean environment for residents.

9. Documenting resident assessments, care plans, interventions, and response to treatments accurately and maintaining proper records.

10. Engaging in ongoing education and professional development to stay updated on the latest advancements in geriatric nursing, gerontology, and long-term care practices.

Degree(s) Required

To become a long-term care nurse, you need to earn a degree in nursing. The two common degree paths are an Associate Degree in Nursing (ADN) or a Bachelor of Science in Nursing (BSN). However, some employers may prefer or require a BSN for long-term care nursing positions due to the comprehensive knowledge and critical thinking skills gained.

Salary
$64,470 - $107,740

Specialty Certifications Available or Needed
Certification in gerontological nursing can demonstrate specialized knowledge and competence in long-term care. The American Nurses Credentialing Center (ANCC) offers the Gerontological Nursing Certification (RN-BC) credential. Eligibility for the RN-BC certification typically requires a combination of education, clinical experience, and the successful completion of an exam.

Job Requirements
Long-term care nursing requires a strong foundation in medical-surgical nursing skills, as well as additional knowledge and skills specific to geriatric care. Job requirements may include:

1. Proficiency in assessing and managing the complex medical needs of older adults, including chronic diseases, cognitive impairments, and age-related changes.
2. Knowledge of geriatric syndromes, such as falls, pressure ulcers, delirium, or polypharmacy, and the ability to implement preventive measures and appropriate interventions.
3. Competence in administering medications and treatments commonly used in long-term care, understanding the unique considerations for older adults, and managing polypharmacy.
4. Skill in assisting with ADLs and providing personal care while promoting residents' autonomy, dignity, and quality of life.
5. Understanding of geriatric mental health issues, including dementia, depression, and anxiety, and the ability to provide appropriate support and interventions.
6. Effective communication and interpersonal skills to interact with residents, their families, and the interdisciplinary team in a compassionate and empathetic manner.
7. Collaboration with the healthcare team, including physicians, therapists, social workers, and dietitians, to provide coordinated care and address residents' physical, emotional, and social needs.
8. Proficiency in documentation and record-keeping, ensuring accurate and complete documentation of resident assessments, care plans, interventions, and responses.

Miscellaneous Information You Should Know

To enter the long-term care nursing specialty, you may consider the following:

1. Gain clinical experience in relevant areas: Acquire experience in geriatric units, nursing homes, assisted living facilities, or rehabilitation centers to develop a foundation in geriatric care, managing chronic conditions, and promoting the well-being of older adults.

2. Develop empathy and effective communication skills: Long-term care nursing requires establishing trusting relationships with residents and their families. Enhance your communication skills to engage with older adults, listen to their concerns, and provide emotional support.

3. Pursue additional education or certifications in gerontological nursing: Consider attending workshops, seminars, or specialized training programs in gerontological nursing to enhance your knowledge and skills. These programs can provide education on geriatric syndromes, age-related changes, geriatric mental health, and person-centered care approaches.

4. Stay updated with evidence-based practices: Keep yourself informed about current research, evidence-based practices, and clinical guidelines related to long-term care and gerontology. Access resources provided by professional organizations, such as the Gerontological Advanced Practice Nurses Association (GAPNA), to stay up-to-date with emerging practices and advancements in the field.

5. Networking and professional involvement: Engage with professional organizations and communities focused on geriatric nursing or long-term care to connect with other long-term care nurses, access educational resources, and stay informed about career opportunities. Participate in conferences, webinars, or local chapter meetings to expand your knowledge and network with professionals in the field.

Remember that specific requirements and preferences may vary depending on the healthcare organization, geographical location, and level of experience desired for long-term care nursing positions.

| Urology Nursing |

Urology Nursing is a specialized field of nursing that focuses on providing care for patients with urological conditions, disorders, and diseases. Urology Nurses work in various healthcare settings, including hospitals, clinics, and urology practices. They assist with diagnostic procedures, provide patient education, administer treatments, and offer support to patients with urological conditions affecting the urinary system, including the kidneys, bladder, ureters, and urethra.

A Day in the Life

A typical day in the life of a Urology Nurse may involve:

1. Patient Assessment: Conducting comprehensive assessments of patients with urological conditions, including obtaining medical histories, performing physical examinations, and assessing symptoms related to urinary problems.

2. Diagnostic Procedures: Assisting urologists during diagnostic procedures such as cystoscopies, urodynamic testing, and prostate biopsies. Preparing patients for procedures, providing education, and assisting with the management of potential complications.

3. Patient Education: Educating patients and their families about urological conditions, treatment options, and self-care measures. Providing instruction on medication management, dietary modifications, and lifestyle changes to promote bladder and urinary health.

4. Catheter Management: Assessing, inserting, monitoring, and managing urinary catheters. Ensuring proper catheter care, preventing infections, and troubleshooting catheter-related issues.

5. Wound Care: Providing wound care for urological surgical patients, including incision site care, dressing changes, and monitoring for signs of infection.

6. Medication Administration: Administering medications, including antibiotics, pain medications, and bladder instillations, as prescribed by urologists. Monitoring patients for adverse reactions and providing appropriate education regarding medication administration and potential side effects.

7. Patient Support: Offering emotional support and counseling to patients and their families as they navigate urological conditions, treatment options, and potential lifestyle adjustments.

8. Collaboration with the Healthcare Team: Collaborating with urologists, surgeons, nurse practitioners, and other healthcare professionals to develop and implement individualized care plans for patients. Communicating and coordinating care to ensure continuity and optimal

outcomes.

9. Continence Management: Assessing and managing urinary incontinence, including implementing bladder retraining programs, prescribing and managing bladder control medications, and recommending behavioral interventions.

10. Documentation: Ensuring accurate and thorough documentation of patient assessments, interventions, and outcomes in medical records. Adhering to legal and ethical standards for documentation.

Degree(s) Required

To become a Urology Nurse, you need to earn a degree in nursing. The two common degree paths are an Associate Degree in Nursing (ADN) or a Bachelor of Science in Nursing (BSN). However, some employers may prefer or require a BSN due to its comprehensive curriculum and broader range of nursing skills.

Salary

$66,640 - $110,930

Specialty Certifications Available or Needed

Obtaining specialty certification in Urology Nursing can validate advanced knowledge and expertise in this field. The Society of Urologic Nurses and Associates (SUNA) offers the Certified Urologic Registered Nurse (CURN) certification, which demonstrates specialized knowledge in urological care. Additionally, the Wound, Ostomy, and Continence Nursing Certification Board (WOCNCB) offers the Certified Continence Care Nurse (CCCN) certification, which focuses on the management of urinary incontinence and bladder disorders.

Job Requirements

Urology Nurses require specific knowledge and skills to provide effective care to patients with urological conditions. Job requirements may include:

1. Urological Knowledge: Acquire a solid understanding of urological anatomy, physiology, and common urological conditions, such as urinary tract infections, kidney stones, prostate disorders, urinary incontinence, and urological cancers.

2. Diagnostic and Procedure Assistance: Familiarity with urological diagnostic procedures and interventions, including cystoscopies, urodynamic testing, prostate biopsies, and placement and management of urinary catheters.

3. Patient Assessment Skills: Proficiency in conducting comprehensive

assessments of patients with urological conditions, including a thorough history, physical examination, and assessment of urinary symptoms.

4. Patient Education: Ability to effectively educate patients and their families about urological conditions, treatment options, medications, and self-care measures to promote optimal urinary health.

5. Continence Management: Competence in managing urinary incontinence, including implementing behavioral interventions, recommending appropriate continence products, and educating patients on bladder retraining techniques.

6. Surgical Assistance: Assisting urologists during surgical procedures, such as transurethral resections, nephrectomies, or prostatectomies. Preparing patients for surgery, providing pre- and post-operative care, and managing potential complications.

7. Collaborative Care: Collaboration with urologists, surgeons, nurse practitioners, and other healthcare professionals to develop and implement individualized care plans for patients. Effective communication and interdisciplinary teamwork are essential.

8. Catheter Management: Competence in urinary catheterization, including assessment, insertion, maintenance, troubleshooting, and preventing catheter-associated urinary tract infections (CAUTIs).

9. Documentation: Ensuring accurate and thorough documentation of patient assessments, interventions, and outcomes in medical records. Adhering to legal and ethical standards for documentation.

10. Continual Learning: Staying updated on current urological research, evidence-based practices, and advancements in urological care through professional development activities, attending conferences, and participating in urology-specific workshops and seminars.

Miscellaneous Information You Should Know

To enter the Urology Nursing specialty, you may consider the following:

1. Gain Clinical Experience: Seek opportunities to work in urology or surgical units during your nursing education or through internships and clinical rotations. This experience will provide exposure to urological conditions, diagnostic procedures, and urological surgeries.

2. Join Professional Organizations: Consider joining professional organizations, such as the Society of Urologic Nurses and Associates (SUNA), to access resources, educational opportunities, and networking events specific to urology nursing.

3. Pursue Continuing Education: Engage in continuing education activities, such as attending urology conferences, workshops, and webinars, to stay updated on advancements and best practices in urological care.

4. Seek Mentorship and Collaboration: Connect with experienced

Urology Nurses or urologists who can serve as mentors and provide guidance as you develop your urology nursing skills.

5. Specialty Training Programs: Explore specialized training programs or fellowships in urology nursing offered by healthcare institutions or professional organizations to enhance your knowledge and skills in this field.

Remember that specific requirements and preferences may vary depending on the employer, healthcare facility, or urology practice where you plan to practice as a Urology Nurse.

| Radiology Nursing |

Radiology nursing, also known as diagnostic imaging nursing, is a specialized field that focuses on providing nursing care to patients undergoing diagnostic and interventional radiology procedures. Radiology nurses work closely with radiologists and radiologic technologists to ensure patient safety, provide comfort, and assist in the imaging process. They work in various healthcare settings, including hospitals, outpatient imaging centers, and radiology departments.

A Day in the Life

A typical day in the life of a radiology nurse may involve:

1. Patient Assessment: Conducting pre-procedure assessments to gather relevant medical history, assess the patient's condition, and ensure the patient is prepared for the radiology procedure.

2. Patient Education: Providing clear and concise explanations of radiology procedures to patients and their families, including what to expect, any necessary preparations, and potential risks or side effects.

3. Patient Preparation: Assisting patients in proper positioning and ensuring they are comfortable during the imaging procedure. Administering medications or contrast agents as directed by the radiologist.

4. Collaboration with Radiologists and Technologists: Working closely with radiologists and radiologic technologists to ensure accurate imaging techniques, including positioning, equipment settings, and image quality.

5. Monitoring Patient Safety: Observing patients during imaging procedures, monitoring vital signs, and assessing for any adverse reactions or complications.

6. Emergency Response: Being prepared to respond to any emergencies or adverse events that may occur during or immediately after a radiology procedure, such as an allergic reaction or contrast extravasation.

7. Documentation and Record-Keeping: Maintaining accurate and detailed documentation of patient assessments, procedures performed, medication administration, and any adverse events or complications.

8. Patient Advocacy: Advocating for patients' rights, ensuring informed consent, and addressing any concerns or questions they may have before, during, or after the procedure.

9. Quality Assurance: Participating in quality improvement initiatives, including monitoring and reporting any safety concerns or incidents related to radiology procedures.

10. Ongoing Education: Staying updated with advancements in radiology technology, safety protocols, and evidence-based practices in radiology nursing through continuing education and professional

development.

Degree(s) Required

To become a radiology nurse, you need to earn a degree in nursing. The two common degree paths are an Associate Degree in Nursing (ADN) or a Bachelor of Science in Nursing (BSN). However, some employers may prefer or require a BSN for radiology nursing positions due to the comprehensive knowledge and critical thinking skills gained.

Salary

$66,640 - $110,930

Specialty Certifications Available or Needed

Certification in radiology nursing can demonstrate specialized knowledge and competence. The Association for Radiologic & Imaging Nursing (ARIN) offers the Certified Radiology Nurse (CRN) credential. Eligibility for the CRN certification typically requires a combination of education, clinical experience in radiology nursing, and successful completion of an exam.

Job Requirements

Radiology nursing requires a strong foundation in nursing practice, as well as additional knowledge and skills specific to radiology and imaging procedures. Job requirements may include:

1. Knowledge of radiology procedures and imaging techniques, including X-rays, computed tomography (CT), magnetic resonance imaging (MRI), ultrasound, and interventional radiology procedures.

2. Understanding of radiation safety protocols and the ability to ensure patient and staff safety during imaging procedures.

3. Proficiency in patient assessment, including identifying contraindications, allergies, and potential risks associated with contrast agents or specific imaging procedures.

4. Familiarity with imaging equipment and technology, including the ability to troubleshoot and assist in equipment setup and calibration.

5. Collaboration with radiologists, radiologic technologists, and other members of the healthcare team to provide comprehensive patient care and ensure accurate imaging results.

6. Excellent communication skills to educate patients and their families about procedures, obtain informed consent, and address any questions or concerns.

7. Ability to provide emotional support to patients who may experience anxiety or discomfort during imaging procedures.

8. Documentation and record-keeping skills to maintain accurate and detailed patient records, including procedural information, medications administered, and any adverse events or complications.

9. Knowledge of emergency response protocols and the ability to act quickly and effectively in emergency situations.

10. Ability to stay updated with current research, evidence-based practices, and clinical guidelines related to radiology nursing.

Miscellaneous Information You Should Know

To enter the radiology nursing specialty, you may consider the following:

1. Gain experience in radiology or imaging settings: Seek opportunities to gain experience in radiology departments, outpatient imaging centers, or interventional radiology units. This experience will provide valuable exposure to the imaging process, radiology procedures, and patient care in a radiology setting.

2. Pursue additional education or certifications in radiology nursing: Consider attending workshops, seminars, or specialized training programs in radiology nursing to enhance your knowledge and skills. These programs can provide education on radiology procedures, contrast administration, radiation safety, and evidence-based practices in radiology nursing.

3. Stay updated with technological advancements: Stay informed about current advancements in radiology technology, imaging techniques, and safety protocols. Regularly access resources provided by professional organizations, such as the Association for Radiologic & Imaging Nursing (ARIN) and the Radiological Society of North America (RSNA), to stay up-to-date with emerging practices and advancements in the field.

4. Networking and professional involvement: Engage with professional organizations and communities focused on radiology nursing to connect with other radiology nurses, access educational resources, and stay informed about career opportunities. Participate in conferences, webinars, or local chapter meetings to expand your knowledge and network with professionals in the field.

Remember that specific requirements and preferences may vary depending on the healthcare organization, geographical location, and level of experience desired for radiology nursing positions.

| Subacute Nursing |

Subacute Nursing is a specialized field of nursing that focuses on the care and rehabilitation of patients who require an intermediate level of care between acute hospitalization and traditional long-term care. Subacute care is designed for patients who are stable but still require skilled nursing and medical interventions. Subacute nurses provide comprehensive care, including medical management, specialized treatments, therapy, and rehabilitation services, to help patients regain their functional abilities and transition to a lower level of care.

A Day in the Life

A typical day in the life of a Subacute Nurse may involve:

1. Assessment and Planning: Conducting comprehensive assessments of patients upon admission, including physical, psychological, and social assessments. Developing individualized care plans in collaboration with the interdisciplinary team to address the patient's specific needs and goals.

2. Medical Management: Administering medications, monitoring vital signs, and managing chronic medical conditions. Collaborating with physicians and other healthcare professionals to coordinate medical interventions and treatments.

3. Skilled Nursing Care: Providing direct care to patients, including wound care, catheter care, tube feedings, and pain management. Ensuring patient comfort, safety, and infection control measures.

4. Rehabilitation and Therapy: Collaborating with physical therapists, occupational therapists, and speech-language pathologists to implement rehabilitation programs and assist patients in regaining their functional abilities, mobility, and independence.

5. Monitoring and Evaluation: Monitoring patients' progress, assessing treatment effectiveness, and adjusting care plans as necessary. Conducting ongoing evaluations and reassessments to track improvements and identify areas requiring further intervention.

6. Patient and Family Education: Providing education to patients and their families regarding their medical condition, treatment plan, self-care techniques, and strategies for managing their health after discharge.

7. Communication and Collaboration: Communicating effectively with patients, their families, and the interdisciplinary team to ensure continuity of care. Participating in team meetings, care conferences, and discharge planning to facilitate a smooth transition to the appropriate level of care.

8. Documentation and Record-Keeping: Maintaining accurate and detailed documentation of patient assessments, care provided, treatment outcomes, and communication with healthcare team members. Adhering to

legal and ethical standards of documentation.

9. Emotional Support: Offering emotional support and empathy to patients and their families during their rehabilitation journey. Assisting patients in coping with their physical limitations, addressing emotional needs, and promoting a positive and supportive environment.

10. Continuous Learning: Engaging in ongoing professional development, staying updated on best practices, new treatments, and advances in subacute nursing care. Participating in relevant training programs, workshops, and conferences to enhance skills and knowledge.

Degree(s) Required

To become a Subacute Nurse, you need to earn a degree in nursing. The two common degree paths are an Associate Degree in Nursing (ADN) or a Bachelor of Science in Nursing (BSN). However, some employers or subacute care facilities may prefer or require a BSN due to the comprehensive knowledge and critical thinking skills gained.

Salary

$64,470 - $107,740

Specialty Certifications Available or Needed

Certification in subacute nursing is not as common as in other specialties. However, some organizations offer certifications related to geriatric care or rehabilitation nursing, which may be applicable to subacute nursing practice. Examples include the Gerontological Nursing Certification (RN-BC) offered by the American Nurses Credentialing Center (ANCC) or the Rehabilitation Nursing Certification (CRRN) offered by the Rehabilitation Nursing Certification Board (RNCB).

Job Requirements

Subacute Nurses require specific knowledge and skills to effectively care for patients in this setting. Job requirements may include:

1. Strong assessment and critical thinking skills to evaluate patients' needs, monitor their condition, and identify any changes or complications.

2. Competence in skilled nursing care, including wound care, medication administration, pain management, and catheter care.

3. Understanding of rehabilitation principles and therapies to assist patients in regaining their functional abilities and independence.

4. Proficiency in coordinating care with various healthcare professionals, including physicians, therapists, social workers, and case managers.

5. Effective communication and interpersonal skills to establish rapport with patients and their families, providing emotional support and education.

6. Documentation and record-keeping skills to maintain accurate and detailed patient records, care plans, and progress notes.

7. Knowledge of infection control practices and ability to implement appropriate measures to prevent the spread of infections in a healthcare setting.

8. Flexibility and adaptability to work with diverse patient populations and handle complex medical conditions.

9. Compassion, patience, and a supportive approach to assist patients in their recovery process.

10. Commitment to continuous learning and staying updated on advancements in subacute care, rehabilitation techniques, and evidence-based practice.

Miscellaneous Information You Should Know

To enter the Subacute Nursing specialty, you may consider the following:

1. Gain experience in relevant healthcare settings: Seek opportunities to gain experience in settings that provide subacute care, such as rehabilitation centers, long-term acute care hospitals, or transitional care units. This experience will provide you with a solid foundation in subacute nursing principles and practices.

2. Obtain certifications or additional training: While certifications specific to subacute nursing may be limited, consider pursuing certifications or additional training in related areas such as geriatrics, rehabilitation nursing, or wound care. These certifications can enhance your skills and knowledge in providing specialized care to subacute patients.

3. Professional networking: Join professional organizations, such as the Association of Rehabilitation Nurses (ARN) or the National Association for Healthcare Quality (NAHQ), to connect with other nurses working in subacute care. Attend conferences, workshops, or webinars to expand your knowledge, gain insights, and stay updated on the latest advancements in subacute nursing.

Remember that specific requirements and preferences may vary depending on the subacute care facility, region, or healthcare organization where you plan to practice as a Subacute Nurse.

| Solid Organ Transplant Nursing |

Solid Organ Transplant Nursing is a specialized field of nursing that focuses on the care and management of patients undergoing solid organ transplantation. This includes the transplantation of organs such as the heart, lungs, liver, kidney, pancreas, and intestines. Solid organ transplant nurses play a crucial role in coordinating pre-transplant evaluations, post-transplant care, immunosuppressive medication management, patient and family education, and ongoing follow-up to support the successful transplantation and long-term well-being of transplant recipients.

A Day in the Life

A typical day in the life of a Solid Organ Transplant Nurse may involve:

1. Pre-Transplant Evaluations: Assessing potential transplant recipients and coordinating pre-transplant evaluations, including laboratory tests, imaging, and consultations with various healthcare professionals to determine transplant eligibility.

2. Patient Education: Providing comprehensive education to transplant candidates and their families regarding the transplantation process, risks, benefits, and the importance of adherence to the prescribed treatment plan.

3. Coordination of Transplant Procedures: Collaborating with the transplant team, including surgeons, anesthesiologists, and other healthcare professionals, to ensure a smooth and safe transplant procedure.

4. Post-Transplant Care: Monitoring transplant recipients closely in the immediate post-transplant period, assessing graft function, managing immunosuppressive medications, and preventing complications such as infections and rejection.

5. Medication Management: Ensuring proper administration and monitoring of immunosuppressive medications, including assessing drug levels, managing side effects, and educating patients about the importance of medication adherence.

6. Collaborative Care: Collaborating with various healthcare professionals, including pharmacists, social workers, dietitians, and physical therapists, to provide comprehensive care and support to transplant recipients.

7. Patient and Family Support: Providing emotional support to patients and their families throughout the transplant journey, addressing their concerns, and facilitating access to support groups or counseling services as needed.

8. Ongoing Follow-Up: Monitoring transplant recipients' long-term outcomes, performing regular assessments, ordering follow-up tests, and coordinating ongoing care to ensure graft function and overall well-being.

9. Education and Research: Staying updated on the latest advancements in transplantation nursing through continuing education, participating in research projects, and contributing to evidence-based practice in the field.

Degree(s) Required

To become a Solid Organ Transplant Nurse, you need to earn a degree in nursing. The two common degree paths are an Associate Degree in Nursing (ADN) or a Bachelor of Science in Nursing (BSN). However, some employers or transplant centers may prefer or require a BSN due to the comprehensive knowledge and critical thinking skills gained.

Salary

$68,450 - $115,800

Specialty Certifications Available or Needed

Certification in Solid Organ Transplant Nursing can demonstrate specialized knowledge and competence in this field. The American Board for Transplant Certification (ABTC) offers the Certified Clinical Transplant Nurse (CCTN) certification. Eligibility for the CCTN certification typically requires a combination of education, clinical experience in solid organ transplantation, and successful completion of an exam.

Job Requirements

Solid Organ Transplant Nurses require specific knowledge and skills to effectively care for transplant patients. Job requirements may include:

1. Comprehensive understanding of the transplantation process, including evaluation, selection criteria, surgical procedures, immunosuppressive medications, and post-transplant care.

2. Knowledge of the specific considerations and potential complications related to various solid organ transplants, such as heart, lung, liver, kidney, pancreas, and intestinal transplantation.

3. Competence in assessing graft function, recognizing signs of rejection or complications, and implementing appropriate interventions.

4. Expertise in managing immunosuppressive medications, including dosing, monitoring drug levels, managing side effects, and educating patients about medication adherence.

5. Understanding of infection prevention strategies and vigilant monitoring for infections, which can pose significant risks to transplant recipients.

6. Ability to provide patient and family education, including pre-transplant education, medication management, lifestyle modifications, and signs of potential complications.

7. Collaboration and communication skills to work effectively with a multidisciplinary transplant team, including surgeons, pharmacists, social workers, dietitians, and other healthcare professionals.

8. Documentation and record-keeping skills to maintain accurate and detailed transplant records, including assessments, medication administration, laboratory results, and follow-up care plans.

9. Compassion and empathy to support patients and their families throughout the transplant journey, including addressing emotional and psychosocial needs.

10. Ongoing professional development to stay updated on advancements in transplantation nursing, including attending conferences, participating in continuing education, and maintaining knowledge of current research and best practices.

Miscellaneous Information You Should Know

To enter the Solid Organ Transplant Nursing specialty, you may consider the following:

1. Gain experience in critical care or specialty units: Acquiring experience in critical care settings, such as the Intensive Care Unit (ICU) or specialty units focused on the care of transplant recipients, can provide valuable knowledge and skills related to complex patient management, acute care interventions, and multi-system organ dysfunction.

2. Seek opportunities for transplantation-focused education and training: Look for professional development opportunities, such as workshops, conferences, or online courses that specifically focus on solid organ transplantation nursing. These educational activities can enhance your understanding of transplantation principles, immunosuppressive medications, and post-transplant care.

3. Network with professionals in the field: Engage with professional organizations, such as the International Transplant Nurses Society (ITNS), to connect with other transplant nurses, access educational resources, and stay updated on the latest research and advancements in solid organ transplantation.

Remember that specific requirements and preferences may vary depending on the transplant center, healthcare facility, or region where you plan to practice as a Solid Organ Transplant Nurse.

| Cruise Ship Nursing |

Cruise Ship Nursing is a unique nursing specialty that involves providing healthcare services to passengers and crew members aboard cruise ships. Cruise Ship Nurses work in collaboration with a healthcare team to deliver medical care, emergency response, health education, and support to individuals on board. They handle a wide range of healthcare needs, from routine medical concerns to emergencies, and ensure the well-being of passengers and crew members throughout the voyage.

A Day in the Life

A typical day in the life of a Cruise Ship Nurse may involve:

1. Medical Clinic Operations: Managing the ship's medical clinic and ensuring it is well-equipped and stocked with necessary medications and supplies.

2. Medical Assessments: Conducting initial health assessments on passengers and crew members who seek medical attention, evaluating their medical history, current health status, and healthcare needs.

3. Medical Care: Providing appropriate medical care and treatment for various illnesses, injuries, and medical conditions encountered on board, such as seasickness, minor injuries, respiratory infections, and gastrointestinal issues.

4. Emergency Response: Responding to medical emergencies on board, coordinating with the ship's emergency response team, and providing immediate medical interventions as needed.

5. Medication Management: Administering medications to patients according to prescribed orders, ensuring accurate dosage, documentation, and following safety protocols.

6. Health Education: Conducting health education sessions for passengers and crew members on topics such as hygiene, disease prevention, and health promotion.

7. Disease Outbreak Control: Collaborating with shipboard public health officials to monitor and control the spread of communicable diseases on the ship, implementing infection control measures, and providing guidance on disease prevention strategies.

8. Coordination with Onshore Medical Facilities: Coordinating with onshore medical facilities and local healthcare providers in case of medical emergencies or the need for specialized care beyond the ship's capabilities.

9. Documentation and Reporting: Maintaining accurate and comprehensive medical records, documenting assessments, treatments, medications administered, and any incidents or encounters.

10. Collaboration with the Ship's Staff: Working closely with the ship's

officers, crew members, and other departments to ensure the overall well-being and safety of passengers and crew members.

11. Continuous Professional Development: Staying updated on current medical practices, advancements, and emergency protocols through ongoing education and professional development activities.

12. Safety and Security: Adhering to safety and security protocols specific to cruise ship operations to maintain a safe environment for passengers, crew members, and oneself.

13. Multicultural Sensitivity: Being culturally sensitive and adapting nursing care to meet the diverse needs of passengers and crew members from different countries and backgrounds.

Degree(s) Required

To become a Cruise Ship Nurse, you need to have a degree in nursing. The two common degree paths are an Associate Degree in Nursing (ADN) or a Bachelor of Science in Nursing (BSN). However, some cruise lines may prefer or require a BSN due to the specialized nature of the role. Additionally, having a strong foundation in medical-surgical nursing, emergency care, and primary care is beneficial.

Salary

$68,450 - $115,800

Specialty Certifications Available or Needed

While not mandatory, obtaining specialty certifications related to cruise ship nursing can demonstrate your expertise and commitment to the field. One recognized certification is:

1. Certification in Travel Health (CTH): Offered by the International Society of Travel Medicine (ISTM), this certification validates your knowledge and skills in providing healthcare to travelers. It covers topics such as travel-related diseases, immunizations, travel safety, and health promotion during travel.

Obtaining the CTH certification can enhance your understanding of travel health considerations and equip you with the necessary knowledge to address the specific healthcare needs of cruise ship passengers and crew members.

Job Requirements

Cruise Ship Nursing requires specific skills and qualities to provide quality care within the unique environment of a cruise ship. Job requirements may include:

1. Clinical Competence: Proficiency in providing a wide range of medical care, emergency response, and primary care services.

2. Emergency and Critical Care Skills: Ability to handle medical emergencies and provide critical care in a maritime environment, often with limited resources and infrastructure.

3. Cultural Competence: Demonstrating cultural competence and sensitivity to work with passengers and crew members from diverse cultural and linguistic backgrounds.

4. Effective Communication: Excellent communication and interpersonal skills to interact with passengers, crew members, and other healthcare professionals on board.

5. Adaptability and Flexibility: Ability to adapt to the unique challenges and dynamics of working on a cruise ship, including long working hours, tight living quarters, and potential seasickness.

6. Multidisciplinary Collaboration: Working collaboratively with the ship's officers, crew members, and other departments to provide comprehensive care and support.

7. Licensing and Certifications: Obtaining and maintaining a valid nursing license in the country of your practice. Complying with any additional licensing or credentialing requirements specific to cruise ship nursing set by your employer or local regulations.

8. Physical Stamina: Being physically fit and having the stamina to navigate the ship, climb stairs, and respond to medical emergencies in potentially challenging conditions.

9. Knowledge of Maritime Regulations: Familiarity with maritime regulations, safety protocols, and emergency procedures to ensure compliance and promote the safety of passengers and crew members.

Miscellaneous Information You Should Know

To enter the Cruise Ship Nursing specialty, consider the following:

1. Obtain Relevant Experience: Gaining experience in emergency care, primary care, travel health, or other acute care settings can provide a strong foundation for working in the cruise ship environment.

2. Training and Orientation: Cruise lines typically provide specialized training and orientation programs for nurses joining their medical teams. This may include shipboard safety procedures, emergency response protocols, and familiarization with onboard medical facilities and equipment.

3. Travel Health Education: Acquiring knowledge and training in travel health, including immunizations, common travel-related illnesses, and health promotion during travel, can be beneficial for working with cruise

ship passengers.

4. Multilingual Skills: Possessing fluency or proficiency in multiple languages can be an advantage in effectively communicating with passengers and crew members from diverse backgrounds.

5. Personal Safety: Adhering to safety protocols and measures on board, including the use of personal protective equipment and following security guidelines.

6. International Travel Requirements: Being aware of any visa requirements, immunization regulations, and health certifications necessary for working on international cruise ships.

7. Flexibility in Schedule and Location: Recognizing that working on a cruise ship often involves being away from home for extended periods and adjusting to a rotational schedule.

Entering the Cruise Ship Nursing specialty offers the opportunity to combine healthcare expertise with a unique travel experience. It requires adaptability, strong clinical skills, effective communication, and a commitment to providing high-quality care in a maritime environment.

| Travel Nursing |

Travel Nursing is a unique nursing specialty that involves temporary assignments in various healthcare facilities across different locations. Travel Nurses work on short-term contracts, typically ranging from 8 to 13 weeks, in hospitals, clinics, and other healthcare settings. They provide patient care, fill staffing needs, and bring their expertise to different healthcare environments. Travel Nursing offers opportunities for adventure, professional growth, and the ability to experience diverse healthcare settings and patient populations.

A Day in the Life

A typical day in the life of a Travel Nurse may involve:

1. Transitioning to a New Location: Traveling to a new location and getting acclimated to the healthcare facility, unit, and the local community.

2. Orientation and Training: Participating in facility-specific orientation and training to familiarize oneself with policies, procedures, electronic health records (EHRs), and unit protocols.

3. Patient Care: Providing direct patient care according to the specific unit's needs and scope of practice. This may involve administering medications, performing assessments, monitoring vital signs, dressing changes, assisting with procedures, and collaborating with the healthcare team.

4. Adapting to Different Environments: Adjusting to different patient populations, healthcare systems, facility protocols, and staffing dynamics in each assignment.

5. Building Relationships: Establishing rapport with patients, families, and the healthcare team to facilitate effective communication, collaboration, and patient-centered care.

6. Documentation: Ensuring accurate and timely documentation of patient assessments, interventions, and outcomes following facility-specific guidelines and EHR systems.

7. Flexibility and Adaptability: Adapting to changing patient needs, varying acuity levels, and the specific workflow of each healthcare facility.

8. Patient Education: Providing patient education on self-care, medication administration, managing chronic conditions, and preparing patients and families for discharge.

9. Collaborative Care: Collaborating with healthcare professionals, including physicians, nurses, therapists, and social workers, to ensure coordinated and comprehensive patient care.

10. Travel and Exploration: Taking advantage of the location by exploring the local area, engaging in recreational activities, and experiencing

different cultures during time off.

Degree(s) Required

To become a Travel Nurse, you need to earn a degree in nursing. The two common degree paths are an Associate Degree in Nursing (ADN) or a Bachelor of Science in Nursing (BSN). While an ADN can provide entry into the field, some travel nursing agencies and healthcare facilities may prefer or require a BSN due to its comprehensive curriculum and broader range of nursing skills.

Salary

$94,250 - $126,810

Specialty Certifications Available or Needed

Specialty certifications are not typically required for travel nursing. However, depending on the assignment and facility, specific certifications may be preferred or required. Examples include Basic Life Support (BLS), Advanced Cardiac Life Support (ACLS), Pediatric Advanced Life Support (PALS), and certifications in specialized areas such as Critical Care (CCRN), Emergency Nursing (CEN), or Labor and Delivery (RNC).

Job Requirements

Travel Nurses require specific skills and qualities to thrive in their role. Job requirements may include:

1. Licensure: Obtain an active Registered Nurse (RN) license in the state(s) where you plan to work as a Travel Nurse. This may involve obtaining a compact nursing license or obtaining individual state licenses, depending on the Nurse Licensure Compact (NLC) regulations.

2. Relevant Experience: Acquire at least one to two years of clinical experience in your chosen specialty before considering travel nursing assignments. This helps build a strong foundation of nursing skills and expertise.

3. Flexibility: Demonstrate flexibility and adaptability to work in various healthcare settings, adjust to different schedules, and adapt to changes in patient populations and clinical environments.

4. Strong Clinical Skills: Possess a solid foundation of clinical skills and competency in your chosen specialty to provide safe and quality patient care independently.

5. Effective Communication: Display excellent communication and interpersonal skills to collaborate with diverse healthcare teams, establish rapport with patients and families quickly, and adapt to new working environments.

6. Organization and Time Management: Demonstrate strong organizational and time management skills to efficiently manage workload, prioritize tasks, and meet the demands of different assignments.

7. Problem-Solving and Critical Thinking: Exhibit strong problem-solving abilities and critical thinking skills to assess complex situations, make sound clinical judgments, and adapt to changing patient conditions.

8. Cultural Competence: Show cultural sensitivity and competence in providing patient-centered care to individuals from diverse backgrounds and communities.

9. Professionalism and Ethics: Uphold the highest standards of professionalism, ethics, and integrity in all aspects of practice, adhering to the Code of Ethics for Nurses.

10. Adaptability to Travel: Be open to travel, including living in temporary housing arrangements and being away from home for extended periods of time.

Miscellaneous Information You Should Know

To enter the Travel Nursing specialty, you may consider the following:

1. Choose a Reputable Travel Nursing Agency: Research and select a reputable travel nursing agency that aligns with your needs and preferences. Look for agencies that offer a wide range of assignments, competitive compensation packages, and comprehensive support services.

2. Obtain Necessary Documentation: Ensure you have all the required documentation, including an active RN license, immunization records, certifications, and professional references.

3. Research Potential Assignments: Research potential assignments and locations that interest you. Consider factors such as cost of living, climate, local amenities, and professional development opportunities.

4. Plan for Housing: Coordinate housing arrangements, whether provided by the agency or independently sourced. Evaluate housing options based on convenience, safety, and affordability.

5. Financial Planning: Understand the financial aspects of travel nursing, including tax implications, travel reimbursements, housing stipends, and healthcare benefits. Seek advice from financial professionals to optimize your financial plan.

6. Professional Networking: Engage in professional networking opportunities, such as attending nursing conferences or joining online communities, to connect with other travel nurses and gain insights into the field.

7. Continuing Education: Seek opportunities for professional development, such as attending workshops, webinars, or obtaining certifications in your specialty. This enhances your skill set and increases

your marketability as a Travel Nurse.

Remember that specific requirements and preferences may vary depending on the travel nursing agency, healthcare facility, or location where you plan to work as a Travel Nurse.

| Plastic Surgery Nursing |

Plastic surgery nursing is a specialized field that focuses on providing healthcare to patients undergoing plastic and reconstructive surgeries. Plastic surgery nurses play a crucial role in assisting surgeons during procedures, educating patients about their surgical options, and providing comprehensive postoperative care. They work in plastic surgery clinics, hospitals, and ambulatory surgical centers, collaborating with plastic surgeons and other healthcare professionals to ensure optimal patient outcomes.

A Day in the Life

A typical day in the life of a plastic surgery nurse may involve:

1. Preoperative Assessments: Conducting preoperative assessments, reviewing medical histories, and ensuring patients are prepared for their surgical procedures.

2. Patient Education: Educating patients about their surgical procedures, including potential risks, benefits, and expected outcomes. Providing instructions for preoperative and postoperative care.

3. Assisting During Procedures: Assisting plastic surgeons during procedures, preparing surgical instruments and supplies, and ensuring the sterile field is maintained.

4. Monitoring Patients: Monitoring patients' vital signs, pain levels, and overall well-being during and after surgery. Managing pain and providing comfort measures.

5. Wound Care: Assisting with wound care, dressing changes, and ensuring proper healing after surgery.

6. Medication Administration: Administering medications, including pain medications and antibiotics, as prescribed by the surgeon.

7. Patient Support: Providing emotional support and reassurance to patients, addressing any concerns or questions they may have.

8. Patient Follow-up: Conducting postoperative assessments and follow-up visits to monitor patients' progress, address any complications, and provide further education and support.

9. Collaboration with the Healthcare Team: Collaborating with plastic surgeons, anesthesiologists, and other healthcare professionals to ensure comprehensive and coordinated care for patients.

10. Ongoing Education: Engaging in continuing education to stay updated on the latest techniques, advancements, and evidence-based practices in plastic surgery nursing.

Degree(s) Required

To become a plastic surgery nurse, you need to earn a degree in nursing. The two common degree paths are an Associate Degree in Nursing (ADN) or a Bachelor of Science in Nursing (BSN). However, some employers may prefer or require a BSN for plastic surgery nursing positions due to the comprehensive knowledge and critical thinking skills gained.

Salary
$66,640 - $110,930

Specialty Certifications Available or Needed
Certification in plastic surgery nursing can demonstrate specialized knowledge and competence. The Plastic Surgical Nursing Certification Board (PSNCB) offers the Certified Plastic Surgical Nurse (CPSN) credential. Eligibility for the CPSN certification typically requires a combination of education, clinical experience in plastic surgery nursing, and successful completion of an exam.

Job Requirements
Plastic surgery nursing requires a strong foundation in nursing practice, as well as additional knowledge and skills specific to plastic surgery care. Job requirements may include:

1. Proficiency in preoperative assessments, including reviewing medical histories, conducting physical examinations, and assessing patients' readiness for surgery.

2. Understanding of various plastic and reconstructive surgical procedures, including cosmetic surgeries, breast reconstructions, facial surgeries, and body contouring procedures.

3. Familiarity with surgical instruments, supplies, and sterile techniques used in plastic surgery procedures.

4. Knowledge of wound care and dressings specific to plastic surgery, including the management of drains and sutures.

5. Effective communication and patient education skills to provide comprehensive information to patients about their surgical procedures, potential risks, and postoperative care instructions.

6. Collaboration with the healthcare team to ensure coordinated care and optimal patient outcomes.

7. Proficiency in documentation and record-keeping, ensuring accurate and thorough documentation of assessments, care plans, interventions, and patient responses.

8. Ability to provide emotional support, empathy, and counseling to patients undergoing plastic surgery procedures.

9. Ability to stay updated with current research, evidence-based

practices, and clinical guidelines related to plastic surgery nursing.

Miscellaneous Information You Should Know

To enter the plastic surgery nursing specialty, you may consider the following:

1. Gain clinical experience in surgical settings: Acquire experience in areas such as operating rooms, surgical units, or outpatient surgical centers to develop a foundation in caring for patients undergoing surgical procedures.

2. Pursue additional education or certifications in plastic surgery nursing: Consider attending workshops, seminars, or specialized training programs in plastic surgery nursing to enhance your knowledge and skills. These programs can provide education on plastic surgery procedures, wound care, patient education, and evidence-based practices in plastic surgery nursing.

3. Stay updated with evidence-based practices: Keep yourself informed about current research, evidence-based practices, and clinical guidelines related to plastic surgery nursing. Access resources provided by professional organizations, such as the International Society of Plastic and Aesthetic Nurses (ISPAN), to stay up-to-date with emerging practices and advancements in the field.

4. Networking and professional involvement: Engage with professional organizations and communities focused on plastic surgery nursing to connect with other plastic surgery nurses, access educational resources, and stay informed about career opportunities. Participate in conferences, webinars, or local chapter meetings to expand your knowledge and network with professionals in the field.

Remember that specific requirements and preferences may vary depending on the healthcare organization, geographical location, and level of experience desired for plastic surgery nursing positions.

| Rheumatology Nursing |

Rheumatology nursing is a specialized field that focuses on providing care to patients with rheumatic diseases, such as rheumatoid arthritis, lupus, osteoarthritis, and fibromyalgia. Rheumatology nurses work closely with rheumatologists and other healthcare professionals to manage the symptoms, promote self-care, and improve the quality of life for patients with rheumatic conditions. They play a crucial role in patient education, medication management, and monitoring disease progression.

A Day in the Life

A typical day in the life of a rheumatology nurse may involve:

1. Patient Assessments: Conducting comprehensive assessments of patients with rheumatic diseases, including evaluating their symptoms, joint function, and overall health status.

2. Medication Management: Educating patients about their prescribed medications, including their purpose, potential side effects, and proper administration. Monitoring medication compliance and assessing the effectiveness of treatments.

3. Disease Education: Providing education to patients and their families about rheumatic diseases, including the nature of the condition, disease management strategies, and lifestyle modifications to enhance overall well-being.

4. Symptom Management: Assisting patients in managing their symptoms, such as pain, joint stiffness, fatigue, and limited mobility. Recommending appropriate strategies, such as exercise, physical therapy, heat or cold therapy, and assistive devices.

5. Collaboration with the Healthcare Team: Collaborating with rheumatologists, physical therapists, occupational therapists, and other healthcare professionals to develop comprehensive care plans tailored to each patient's needs.

6. Patient Support: Offering emotional support and counseling to patients who may experience challenges related to their condition, such as emotional distress, lifestyle adjustments, or social impact.

7. Patient Advocacy: Advocating for patients' rights and needs, ensuring they receive appropriate healthcare services, and facilitating access to resources and support groups.

8. Disease Monitoring: Monitoring disease progression through regular assessments, laboratory tests, and imaging studies. Keeping track of disease activity and adjusting treatment plans as necessary.

9. Documentation and Record-Keeping: Maintaining accurate and up-to-date patient records, including assessments, treatment plans, medication

administration, and disease progress notes.

10. Ongoing Education: Engaging in continuous learning and professional development to stay updated on the latest advancements, research findings, and evidence-based practices in rheumatology nursing.

Degree(s) Required
To become a rheumatology nurse, you need to earn a degree in nursing. The two common degree paths are an Associate Degree in Nursing (ADN) or a Bachelor of Science in Nursing (BSN). However, some employers may prefer or require a BSN for rheumatology nursing positions due to the comprehensive knowledge and critical thinking skills gained.

Salary
$70,670 - $120,690

Specialty Certifications Available or Needed
While there are no specific certifications exclusively for rheumatology nursing, nurses may consider obtaining certifications in related fields to enhance their knowledge and expertise. For example, the Rheumatology Nursing Certification Board (RNCB) offers the Certified Rheumatology Nurse (CRN) credential. Eligibility for the CRN certification typically requires a combination of education, clinical experience in rheumatology nursing, and successful completion of an exam.

Job Requirements
Rheumatology nursing requires a strong foundation in nursing practice, as well as additional knowledge and skills specific to rheumatic diseases. Job requirements may include:

1. Knowledge of rheumatic diseases and their manifestations, including rheumatoid arthritis, lupus, osteoarthritis, and other related conditions.
2. Understanding of diagnostic methods and laboratory tests commonly used in rheumatology, such as blood tests, imaging studies, and joint aspiration.
3. Proficiency in medication management, including knowledge of various disease-modifying antirheumatic drugs (DMARDs), biologics, and immunosuppressants commonly used in the treatment of rheumatic diseases.
4. Competence in patient assessment and the ability to differentiate between different types of arthritis and other rheumatic conditions.
5. Familiarity with symptom management strategies, such as pain management techniques, joint protection, and adaptive aids.
6. Collaboration and communication skills to work effectively with

rheumatologists, physical therapists, occupational therapists, and other members of the healthcare team.

7. Ability to provide patient education and counseling on disease management, treatment options, medication side effects, and self-care techniques.

8. Documentation and record-keeping skills to maintain accurate and detailed patient records, including assessments, treatment plans, medication administration, and disease progress notes.

9. Ability to stay updated with current research, evidence-based practices, and clinical guidelines related to rheumatology nursing.

Miscellaneous Information You Should Know

To enter the rheumatology nursing specialty, you may consider the following:

1. Gain clinical experience in rheumatology settings: Seek opportunities to gain experience in rheumatology clinics, specialty hospitals, or rheumatology departments within larger healthcare organizations. This experience will provide valuable exposure to rheumatic diseases, diagnostic methods, treatment modalities, and patient care in the rheumatology specialty.

2. Pursue additional education or certifications in rheumatology nursing: While there are no specific certifications exclusively for rheumatology nursing, consider attending conferences, workshops, or specialized training programs related to rheumatology care. These educational opportunities can provide in-depth knowledge and skills specific to rheumatic diseases and their management.

3. Networking and professional involvement: Engage with professional organizations, such as the Rheumatology Nurses Society (RNS), to connect with other rheumatology nurses, access educational resources, and stay informed about career opportunities. Participate in conferences, webinars, or local chapter meetings to expand your knowledge and network with professionals in the field.

Remember that specific requirements and preferences may vary depending on the healthcare organization, geographical location, and level of experience desired for rheumatology nursing positions.

| Ophthalmic Nursing |

Ophthalmic nursing is a specialized field that focuses on providing care to patients with eye conditions and diseases. Ophthalmic nurses work in various healthcare settings, including ophthalmology clinics, eye hospitals, surgical centers, and optometry practices. They play a crucial role in assessing, diagnosing, treating, and supporting patients with eye disorders. Ophthalmic nurses provide direct patient care, perform diagnostic tests, assist with eye surgeries, educate patients and their families, and collaborate with ophthalmologists and other eye care professionals.

A Day in the Life
A typical day in the life of an ophthalmic nurse may involve:

1. Assisting with ophthalmic examinations and diagnostic tests, such as visual acuity tests, tonometry, slit-lamp examinations, and fundoscopy.
2. Administering eye medications and performing eye drops instillation, ensuring proper technique and dosage accuracy.
3. Educating patients on eye care, including proper use of contact lenses, eye hygiene, and the importance of regular eye examinations.
4. Assisting ophthalmologists with surgical procedures, such as cataract surgeries, laser surgeries, corneal transplants, or glaucoma procedures.
5. Providing pre-operative and post-operative care to patients undergoing eye surgeries, including administering medications, monitoring vital signs, and assessing surgical site healing.
6. Collaborating with the interdisciplinary healthcare team, including ophthalmologists, optometrists, technicians, and ophthalmic assistants, to provide comprehensive eye care.
7. Assisting in patient education, counseling, and support for those with visual impairments or eye-related chronic conditions.
8. Managing eye emergencies, such as foreign body removal, eye injuries, or acute eye infections, and providing immediate care and treatment.
9. Conducting ophthalmic research, participating in clinical trials, and staying updated on the latest advancements in ophthalmology and eye care.
10. Engaging in ongoing education and professional development to stay updated on the latest advancements in ophthalmic nursing, evidence-based practices, and eye care treatments.

Degree(s) Required
To become an ophthalmic nurse, you need to earn a degree in nursing. The two common degree paths are an Associate Degree in Nursing (ADN) or a Bachelor of Science in Nursing (BSN). However, some employers may prefer or require a BSN for ophthalmic nursing positions due to the

comprehensive knowledge and critical thinking skills gained.

Salary
$66,640 - $110,930

Specialty Certifications Available or Needed
Certification in ophthalmic nursing can demonstrate specialized knowledge and competence. The National Certifying Board for Ophthalmic Registered Nurses (NCBORN) offers the Certified Ophthalmic Registered Nurse (CORNE) credential. Eligibility for the CORNE certification typically requires a combination of education, clinical experience in ophthalmic nursing, and successful completion of an exam.

Job Requirements
Ophthalmic nursing requires a strong foundation in nursing practice, as well as additional knowledge and skills specific to eye care. Job requirements may include:

1. Proficiency in performing ophthalmic examinations and tests, including knowledge of ocular anatomy, visual assessment, and diagnostic procedures.
2. Understanding of common eye conditions and diseases, such as cataracts, glaucoma, macular degeneration, diabetic retinopathy, and refractive errors.
3. Familiarity with ophthalmic medications, including their actions, indications, contraindications, and potential side effects.
4. Effective communication and patient education skills to provide comprehensive information to patients and their families about eye conditions, treatment options, and post-procedure care.
5. Collaboration with the healthcare team, including ophthalmologists, optometrists, technicians, and ophthalmic assistants, to provide coordinated and patient-centered care.
6. Proficiency in documentation and record-keeping, ensuring accurate and complete documentation of patient assessments, treatment plans, interventions, and responses.
7. Ability to adapt to a dynamic and often fast-paced environment, handle emergencies or complications related to eye conditions, and make critical decisions to ensure patient safety and well-being.
8. Knowledge of ocular surgeries and procedures, including pre-operative and post-operative care, surgical asepsis, and sterile techniques.
9. Ability to provide emotional support, empathy, and counseling to patients and their families dealing with vision loss, chronic eye conditions, or the need for eye surgeries.

10. Ability to stay updated with current research, evidence-based practices, and clinical guidelines related to ophthalmic nursing.

Miscellaneous Information You Should Know

To enter the ophthalmic nursing specialty, you may consider the following:

1. Gain clinical experience in ophthalmology or related areas: Acquire experience in ophthalmology clinics, eye hospitals, or surgical centers to develop a foundation in managing patients with eye conditions, understanding ophthalmic examinations, and assisting in eye surgeries.

2. Pursue additional education or certifications in ophthalmic nursing: Consider attending workshops, seminars, or specialized training programs in ophthalmic nursing to enhance your knowledge and skills. These programs can provide education on eye care, ocular assessments, ophthalmic medications, and evidence-based practices in ophthalmology.

3. Stay updated with evidence-based practices: Keep yourself informed about current research, evidence-based practices, and clinical guidelines related to ophthalmic nursing. Access resources provided by professional organizations, such as the American Society of Ophthalmic Registered Nurses (ASORN), to stay up-to-date with emerging practices and advancements in the field.

4. Networking and professional involvement: Engage with professional organizations and communities focused on ophthalmic nursing to connect with other ophthalmic nurses, access educational resources, and stay informed about career opportunities. Participate in conferences, webinars, or local chapter meetings to expand your knowledge and network with professionals in the field.

Remember that specific requirements and preferences may vary depending on the healthcare organization, geographical location, and level of experience desired for ophthalmic nursing positions.

| Trauma Nursing |

Trauma Nursing is a specialized field of nursing that focuses on caring for patients who have experienced traumatic injuries or are in critical condition due to accidents, violence, or medical emergencies. Trauma Nurses work in various healthcare settings, including emergency departments, trauma centers, and intensive care units, where they provide immediate and comprehensive care to stabilize and manage patients with life-threatening injuries.

A Day in the Life

A typical day in the life of a Trauma Nurse may involve:

1. Emergency Response: Responding to trauma alerts and participating in the rapid assessment and management of critically injured patients. Collaborating with a multidisciplinary team to provide immediate life-saving interventions, such as airway management, intravenous access, and hemorrhage control.

2. Patient Assessment: Conducting thorough assessments of patients' injuries, including physical examination, vital sign monitoring, and obtaining a detailed medical history. Assessing and prioritizing injuries based on severity and potential life-threatening conditions.

3. Diagnostic Testing: Coordinating and facilitating diagnostic tests, such as X-rays, CT scans, and laboratory work, to identify additional injuries and guide treatment decisions.

4. Surgical Assistance: Assisting the surgical team during emergency procedures, such as exploratory laparotomy, fracture fixation, or other necessary interventions.

5. Medication Administration: Administering medications, including pain management, antibiotics, and intravenous fluids, as prescribed by the healthcare team. Ensuring proper medication dosages and monitoring for adverse reactions.

6. Wound Care and Dressing Changes: Providing meticulous wound care, including cleaning, debridement, and dressing changes, to prevent infection and promote healing.

7. Monitoring and Critical Care: Monitoring patients' vital signs, cardiac rhythm, oxygenation, and neurological status continuously. Recognizing and responding to changes in patients' conditions promptly and initiating appropriate interventions.

8. Collaborative Care: Collaborating with the trauma team, including physicians, surgeons, respiratory therapists, and social workers, to develop and implement individualized care plans for patients. Participating in interdisciplinary rounds to discuss patient progress and plan ongoing care.

9. Family Support: Providing emotional support and education to patients' families, keeping them informed about their loved one's condition and involving them in the decision-making process.

10. Documentation: Ensuring accurate and timely documentation of patient assessments, interventions, medications administered, and response to treatment. Adhering to legal and ethical standards for documentation.

Degree(s) Required

To become a Trauma Nurse, you need to earn a degree in nursing. The two common degree paths are an Associate Degree in Nursing (ADN) or a Bachelor of Science in Nursing (BSN). However, some employers or trauma centers may prefer or require a BSN due to the comprehensive knowledge and critical thinking skills gained.

Salary

$68,450 - $115,800

Specialty Certifications Available or Needed

Obtaining specialty certification in Trauma Nursing can demonstrate advanced knowledge and expertise in caring for trauma patients. The Board of Certification for Emergency Nursing (BCEN) offers the Trauma Certified Registered Nurse (TCRN) certification, which validates specialized knowledge in trauma nursing.

Job Requirements

Trauma Nurses require specific knowledge and skills to effectively care for patients with traumatic injuries. Job requirements may include:

1. Solid understanding of trauma physiology and pathophysiology: Familiarity with mechanisms of injury, injury patterns, and the body's response to trauma. Knowledge of managing hemorrhage, shock, fractures, head injuries, spinal cord injuries, and other trauma-related conditions.

2. Proficiency in rapid assessment and prioritization: Ability to perform systematic and comprehensive assessments of trauma patients, identify life-threatening injuries, and prioritize interventions accordingly.

3. Competence in trauma resuscitation: Proficiency in advanced cardiac life support (ACLS), advanced trauma life support (ATLS), and other trauma resuscitation protocols. Ability to manage airways, perform chest compressions, insert intravenous lines, and administer fluids and medications during resuscitation efforts.

4. Effective communication and collaboration: Strong communication skills to interact with the trauma team, patients, and their families. Ability to provide clear and concise information, facilitate effective handovers, and

work collaboratively in a high-stress environment.

5. Critical thinking and decision-making: Ability to analyze complex situations, anticipate potential complications, and make quick and appropriate decisions in high-pressure and time-sensitive situations.

6. Adherence to protocols and evidence-based practice: Knowledge of trauma guidelines, protocols, and evidence-based practices. Staying updated on current advancements and research in trauma care.

7. Physical and emotional resilience: Possessing the physical stamina and emotional resilience to handle the physical demands and emotional stress associated with caring for critically injured patients.

8. Effective time management and organizational skills: Ability to prioritize tasks, manage multiple patients simultaneously, and efficiently document patient care activities.

9. Continuous learning and professional development: Commitment to ongoing learning, attending trauma-related workshops, conferences, and seeking opportunities for professional growth in the field of trauma nursing.

Miscellaneous Information You Should Know

To enter the Trauma Nursing specialty, you may consider the following:

1. Acquire experience in an acute care setting: Seek opportunities to work in emergency departments, critical care units, or trauma centers during your nursing education or through internships and clinical rotations. This experience will provide exposure to trauma patients and familiarize you with the fast-paced nature of trauma care.

2. Obtain Advanced Cardiac Life Support (ACLS) certification: ACLS certification is often required or preferred for nurses working in trauma settings. Consider obtaining this certification to enhance your knowledge of cardiac resuscitation and improve your readiness for emergency situations.

3. Pursue Trauma Nursing Core Course (TNCC) training: The TNCC program is designed to provide nurses with essential knowledge and skills in trauma nursing.

4. Seek opportunities for continuing education: Stay updated on trauma care guidelines, research, and advances by engaging in continuing education activities, attending trauma conferences, and participating in trauma-specific workshops and seminars.

5. Develop teamwork and communication skills: Trauma care involves close collaboration with a multidisciplinary team including physicians, surgeons, respiratory therapists, and other healthcare professionals.

Remember that specific requirements and preferences may vary depending on the employer, trauma center, or region where you plan to practice as a Trauma Nurse.

| Dermatology Nursing |

Dermatology nursing focuses on providing specialized care for patients with various dermatological conditions, such as skin diseases, disorders, infections, and injuries. Dermatology nurses work closely with dermatologists and other healthcare professionals to assess, diagnose, and treat skin conditions. They provide patient education, perform skin assessments, administer treatments, and assist with dermatological procedures.

A Day in the Life

A day in the life of a dermatology nurse may involve the following activities:

1. Patient Assessments: Conducting comprehensive skin assessments to identify dermatological conditions and develop treatment plans.

2. Skin Procedures: Assisting dermatologists in performing skin biopsies, mole removals, and other dermatological procedures.

3. Wound Care: Providing specialized wound care for patients with skin injuries or post-surgical wounds.

4. Patient Education: Educating patients on skincare routines, sun protection, and managing skin conditions.

5. Medication Administration: Administering topical and oral medications as prescribed by the dermatologist.

6. Cosmetic Procedures: Assisting with cosmetic procedures such as Botox injections and laser treatments.

7. Collaborative Care: Collaborating with the medical team to provide comprehensive care to patients with skin conditions related to underlying health issues.

8. Record Keeping: Maintaining detailed and accurate medical records of patient assessments, treatments, and progress.

Degree(s) Required

To become a dermatology nurse, you need to earn a degree in nursing. The two common degree paths are an Associate Degree in Nursing (ADN) or a Bachelor of Science in Nursing (BSN). However, pursuing a Bachelor's degree is increasingly preferred in dermatology nursing due to the comprehensive knowledge and critical thinking skills gained. Additionally, obtaining a Master of Science in Nursing (MSN) or a Doctor of Nursing Practice (DNP) can provide advanced training and career opportunities in

138

this field.

Salary
$66,640 - $110,930

Specialty Certifications Available or Needed
Certification in dermatology nursing can demonstrate specialized knowledge and expertise. The Dermatology Nursing Certification Board (DNCB) offers the Dermatology Certified Nurse (DCN) credential. Eligibility for the DCN certification typically requires a combination of education, clinical experience, and the successful completion of an exam.

Job Requirements
Dermatology nursing requires strong clinical skills, knowledge of dermatological conditions and treatments, and the ability to provide compassionate patient care. Job requirements may include:

1. Proficiency in performing skin assessments and identifying various dermatological conditions.
2. Knowledge of dermatological treatments, including medications, topical therapies, and procedures such as biopsies, cryotherapy, or laser therapy.
3. Skill in providing patient education on skin care, prevention, and self-management of dermatological conditions.
4. Competence in assisting with dermatological procedures and minor surgeries.
5. Effective communication skills to interact with patients, families, and healthcare professionals in a dermatology setting.
6. Ability to document patient information accurately and maintain proper record-keeping.

Miscellaneous Information You Should Know
To enter the dermatology nursing specialty, you may consider the following:

1. Gain experience in dermatology or related fields: Acquiring experience in dermatology clinics, dermatology departments, or related areas such as wound care or medical-surgical units can provide a foundation for dermatology nursing. Seek opportunities to work with patients who have skin-related conditions to develop knowledge and skills in dermatology care.
2. Pursue additional education or certifications: Consider pursuing additional education or certifications specific to dermatology nursing. This

may include continuing education courses, workshops, or certificate programs focused on dermatology nursing. These opportunities can enhance your expertise and demonstrate commitment to the specialty.

3. Stay updated with dermatology advancements: Keep yourself informed about new treatments, procedures, and research in dermatology nursing. Access resources provided by professional organizations like the Dermatology Nurses' Association (DNA) or attend dermatology conferences and seminars to stay updated on emerging practices and advancements.

4. Develop strong patient education skills: Patient education is a crucial aspect of dermatology nursing. Enhance your communication and teaching skills to effectively educate patients about their skin conditions, treatment plans, and preventive measures. Familiarize yourself with reputable resources and materials to provide patients with accurate and reliable information.

5. Networking and professional involvement: Engage with professional organizations like the Dermatology Nurses' Association (DNA) to connect with dermatology nurses and professionals in the field. Networking can provide opportunities for mentorship, collaboration, and staying informed about job opportunities or industry trends.

Remember that specific requirements and preferences may vary depending on the healthcare organization, geographical location, and level of experience desired for dermatology nursing positions.

| Sexual Assault Nurse Examiner (SANE) |

Sexual Assault Nurse Examiners (SANEs) are registered nurses with specialized training in providing comprehensive care to individuals who have experienced sexual assault or abuse. SANEs play a critical role in the assessment, documentation, and collection of forensic evidence, as well as providing compassionate care, support, and referrals for survivors of sexual violence. They work collaboratively with law enforcement, forensic professionals, victim advocates, and healthcare teams to ensure the physical and emotional well-being of survivors.

A Day in the Life

A typical day in the life of a Sexual Assault Nurse Examiner may involve:

1. On-call Shifts: SANEs often work on an on-call basis, responding to sexual assault cases when they occur. This can involve being available during evenings, weekends, and holidays to provide timely care and support to survivors.

2. Forensic Evidence Collection: Conducting thorough forensic examinations, which may include gathering evidence from the survivor's body, documenting injuries, and collecting samples for laboratory analysis.

3. Trauma-Informed Care: Providing compassionate and trauma-informed care to survivors, ensuring their physical and emotional comfort throughout the examination process. Offering emotional support, crisis intervention, and resources for ongoing care and healing.

4. Medical Evaluation: Assessing and documenting physical injuries, infections, and other medical concerns related to the assault. Administering necessary medications, such as prophylactic treatment for sexually transmitted infections and emergency contraception.

5. Collaboration with Multidisciplinary Teams: Collaborating with law enforcement, victim advocates, forensic experts, and other healthcare professionals to coordinate care, ensure the preservation of evidence, and support the survivor's legal needs.

6. Documentation and Reporting: Completing accurate and detailed documentation of findings, observations, and procedures in compliance with legal and medical requirements. Maintaining confidentiality and following appropriate chain-of-custody protocols for forensic evidence.

7. Testimony and Legal Proceedings: Providing expert testimony in legal proceedings, when necessary, regarding the findings from the forensic examination. Collaborating with legal professionals to ensure accurate interpretation and presentation of medical evidence.

8. Education and Outreach: Participating in community education and

prevention programs related to sexual violence. Collaborating with local organizations, schools, and healthcare providers to raise awareness and promote resources for survivors.

9. Ongoing Training and Professional Development: Engaging in continuous learning and staying updated on best practices, evidence-based protocols, and emerging research in the field of forensic nursing and sexual assault care.

Degree(s) Required

To become a Sexual Assault Nurse Examiner, you need to earn a degree in nursing. The two common degree paths are an Associate Degree in Nursing (ADN) or a Bachelor of Science in Nursing (BSN). However, some employers or jurisdictions may require or prefer a BSN for SANE positions due to the comprehensive knowledge and critical thinking skills gained.

Salary

$66,650 - $112,470

Specialty Certifications Available or Needed

Certification in forensic nursing or as a Sexual Assault Nurse Examiner (SANE) can demonstrate specialized knowledge and competence in this field. The International Association of Forensic Nurses (IAFN) offers the SANE certification, including several specialized certifications such as Adult/Adolescent SANE, Pediatric SANE, and SANE-A (for SANE-A/Pediatric SANE) or SANE-P (for SANE-P/Adult/Adolescent SANE). Certification requirements typically include a combination of education, clinical experience, and successful completion of an exam.

Job Requirements

Sexual Assault Nurse Examiners require specific knowledge and skills to effectively perform their role. Job requirements may include:

1. Knowledge of forensic nursing practices, including evidence collection, documentation, and chain-of-custody procedures specific to sexual assault cases.

2. Understanding of the dynamics of sexual violence, trauma-informed care, and the psychological impact on survivors.

3. Proficiency in conducting comprehensive physical assessments, documenting injuries, and collecting evidence following established protocols.

4. Familiarity with medical treatments and medications related to sexual assault, including prophylactic treatment for sexually transmitted infections,

emergency contraception, and pregnancy testing.

5. Collaboration and communication skills to work effectively with multidisciplinary teams, including law enforcement, victim advocates, and forensic experts.

6. Ability to provide compassionate and non-judgmental care to survivors of sexual violence, ensuring their physical and emotional well-being throughout the examination process.

7. Ethical and legal understanding of patient confidentiality, mandatory reporting, and maintaining the integrity of forensic evidence.

8. Documentation and record-keeping skills to maintain accurate and detailed documentation of findings, observations, procedures, and evidence.

9. Strong interpersonal and communication skills to support survivors, provide education, and collaborate with legal professionals when necessary.

10. Ability to handle emotionally challenging situations with empathy, sensitivity, and self-care strategies.

Miscellaneous Information You Should Know

To enter the Sexual Assault Nurse Examiner specialty, you may consider the following:

1. Gain clinical experience in emergency, forensic, or women's health settings: Seek opportunities to gain clinical experience in settings that provide exposure to sexual assault care, such as emergency departments, forensic nursing units, or women's health clinics. This experience will provide valuable knowledge and skills in trauma-informed care, evidence collection, and working with survivors of violence.

2. Pursue additional education or certifications in forensic nursing: While certification as a Sexual Assault Nurse Examiner (SANE) is not always mandatory, it can enhance your knowledge and credibility. Consider pursuing certifications such as the SANE certification offered by the International Association of Forensic Nurses (IAFN). Additionally, advanced degrees or courses in forensic nursing or forensic science can provide further specialization.

3. Network with professionals in the field: Engage with professional organizations, such as the International Association of Forensic Nurses (IAFN), to connect with other SANE nurses, access educational resources, and stay updated on the latest research and advancements in the field of forensic nursing.

Remember that specific requirements and preferences may vary depending on the jurisdiction, healthcare facility, or legal system in which you plan to practice as a Sexual Assault Nurse Examiner.

PART II:

NON-CLINICAL SPECIALTIES

| Case Management Nursing |

Case management nursing involves coordinating and managing healthcare services for patients across different care settings. Case managers work closely with patients, healthcare providers, and insurance companies to ensure the delivery of efficient, cost-effective, and high-quality care. They assess patients' needs, develop care plans, coordinate services, and advocate for the patients' best interests.

A Day in the Life
A typical day in the life of a Case Management Nurse may involve:

1. Collaborating with healthcare providers to assess patients' needs and develop individualized care plans.
2. Coordinating services such as medical treatments, therapies, home care, and social services to support the patient's overall well-being.
3. Communicating with patients and their families to provide education on treatment plans and self-management techniques.
4. Advocating for patients and ensuring they have access to appropriate resources and services.
5. Monitoring patients' progress and outcomes and adjusting care plans as needed.
6. Assisting in discharge planning and facilitating transitions of care from one healthcare setting to another.
7. Ensuring continuity of care and minimizing healthcare costs by avoiding unnecessary readmissions and medical services.
8. Collaborating with insurance companies and other payers, such as Medicaid and Medicare, to obtain necessary authorizations for medical treatments and services.
9. Keeping accurate and up-to-date documentation of patient assessments, care plans, and interventions.

Degree(s) Required
To become a case management nurse, you need to earn a degree in nursing. The two common degree paths are an Associate Degree in Nursing (ADN) or a Bachelor of Science in Nursing (BSN). However, pursuing a Bachelor's degree is becoming increasingly preferred in case management roles. Additionally, pursuing higher education, such as a Master of Science in Nursing (MSN) with a specialization in case management or healthcare administration, can enhance your knowledge and advance your career in this field.

Salary
$66,650 - $98,500

Specialty Certifications Available or Needed
Certification in case management nursing can demonstrate specialized knowledge and expertise. The Commission for Case Manager Certification (CCMC) offers the Certified Case Manager (CCM) credential, which is highly recognized in the field. Eligibility for the CCM certification typically requires a combination of education and professional experience in case management.

Job Requirements
Case management nursing requires strong organizational and communication skills, as well as the ability to work collaboratively with various healthcare professionals. Job requirements may include:

1. Proficiency in conducting comprehensive patient assessments, including physical, psychosocial, and environmental factors.
2. Skill in developing individualized care plans based on patients' needs and available resources.
3. Knowledge of healthcare regulations, insurance policies, and reimbursement processes.
4. Ability to coordinate and facilitate healthcare services, including referrals, appointments, and follow-ups.
5. Competence in providing patient education and promoting self-management strategies.
6. Effective communication and collaboration with patients, families, healthcare providers, and insurance companies.

Miscellaneous Information You Should Know
To enter the case management nursing specialty, you may consider the following:

1. Gain experience in diverse healthcare settings: Acquiring experience in various healthcare settings, such as hospitals, clinics, or home health agencies, can provide a broad understanding of the healthcare system and the different aspects of patient care. This diverse experience can be valuable in case management roles.
2. Pursue case management education or certifications: Consider pursuing additional education or certifications specific to case management nursing. These may include a Master's degree or a certificate program in case management. Such programs can provide specialized knowledge and enhance your qualifications in this field.

3. Stay updated with healthcare policies and regulations: Case managers must stay updated with evolving healthcare policies, regulations, and insurance requirements. Actively seek information through professional organizations, journals, and continuing education programs focused on case management.

4. Develop strong communication and advocacy skills: Effective communication and advocacy are essential in case management nursing. Strengthen your communication skills to collaborate with patients, families, and the healthcare team. Advocate for patients' needs, ensuring they receive appropriate and timely care.

5. Networking and professional development: Engage with professional organizations such as the Case Management Society of America (CMSA) to connect with case management professionals, access educational resources, and stay informed about industry trends. Networking can provide valuable insights and potential job opportunities.

Remember that specific requirements and preferences may vary depending on the healthcare organization, geographical location, and level of experience desired for case management nursing positions.

| Family Practice Nursing |

Family practice nursing involves providing comprehensive primary care to individuals and families across the lifespan. Family practice nurses work in outpatient settings, such as family medicine clinics or community health centers. They focus on health promotion, disease prevention, and the management of common acute and chronic conditions. Family practice nurses develop long-term relationships with patients, provide holistic care, and coordinate with other healthcare professionals to address patients' physical, emotional, and social needs.

A Day in the Life

A typical day in the life of a family practice nurse may involve:

1. Conducting patient assessments, including medical history reviews, physical examinations, and screenings.
2. Diagnosing and managing common acute illnesses, such as respiratory infections, injuries, or gastrointestinal disorders.
3. Managing chronic conditions, such as diabetes, hypertension, asthma, or arthritis, by monitoring patients' progress, adjusting medications, and providing patient education.
4. Administering vaccinations, conducting health promotion activities, and providing preventive care, such as cancer screenings or well-child visits.
5. Collaborating with the healthcare team, including physicians, nurse practitioners, and specialists, to develop and implement individualized care plans.
6. Ordering and interpreting diagnostic tests, such as laboratory work or imaging studies, and making appropriate referrals when necessary.
7. Providing patient education on self-care practices, medication management, healthy lifestyle choices, and disease prevention.
8. Documenting patient encounters, maintaining accurate medical records, and ensuring confidentiality of patient information.
9. Engaging in health promotion and community outreach activities, such as health fairs or educational presentations.
10. Staying updated on evidence-based practices, guidelines, and advancements in family practice nursing through continuing education and professional development.

Degree(s) Required

To become a family practice nurse, you need to earn a degree in nursing. The two common degree paths are an Associate Degree in Nursing (ADN) or a Bachelor of Science in Nursing (BSN). However, pursuing a BSN is increasingly preferred for family practice nursing positions due to the comprehensive knowledge and critical thinking skills gained. Additionally, obtaining advanced education, such as a Master of Science in Nursing (MSN) with a specialization in family practice or becoming a Nurse Practitioner (NP), can provide advanced training and expanded responsibilities in this field.

Salary
$63,540 - $109,820

Specialty Certifications Available or Needed
Certification in family practice nursing can demonstrate specialized knowledge and competence. The American Nurses Credentialing Center (ANCC) offers the Family Nurse Practitioner-Board Certified (FNP-BC) credential. Eligibility for the FNP-BC certification typically requires a combination of education, clinical experience, and the successful completion of an exam. It's important to note that certification requirements may vary depending on the role and level of responsibility as a family practice nurse.

Job Requirements
Family practice nursing requires a broad range of clinical skills, strong interpersonal skills, and the ability to provide patient-centered care. Job requirements may include:

1. Proficiency in performing comprehensive assessments, including history taking, physical examinations, and interpreting diagnostic tests.
2. Knowledge of common acute and chronic conditions encountered in family practice, including their diagnosis, treatment, and management.
3. Competence in providing patient education on preventive care, healthy lifestyle choices, and chronic disease management.
4. Skill in performing procedures commonly done in family practice settings, such as wound care, minor suturing, or casting.
5. Effective communication skills to build therapeutic relationships, listen to patient concerns, and collaborate with individuals and families in shared decision-making.
6. Collaboration with the healthcare team, including physicians, nurse practitioners, specialists, and other allied healthcare professionals, to provide comprehensive care.
7. Ability to prioritize patient needs, manage multiple tasks, and work efficiently in a fast-paced environment.
8. Proficiency in documenting patient encounters, maintaining accurate medical records, and adhering to regulatory requirements and confidentiality guidelines.

Miscellaneous Information You Should Know

To enter the family practice nursing specialty, you may consider the following:

1. Gain experience in primary care or ambulatory settings: Acquiring experience in primary care settings, such as family medicine clinics, community health centers, or outpatient departments, can provide a foundation for family practice nursing. Seek opportunities to work with diverse patient populations and develop skills in primary care assessments and interventions.

2. Pursue additional education or certifications: Consider pursuing advanced education, such as a Master's degree with a specialization in family practice nursing or becoming a Nurse Practitioner (NP) with a family practice focus. These advanced degrees can provide additional knowledge and expanded responsibilities in family practice nursing.

3. Enhance communication and patient education skills: Effective communication and patient education are crucial in family practice nursing. Enhance your communication skills to effectively engage with patients, families, and healthcare professionals. Develop patient education strategies to empower individuals and families in managing their health and making informed decisions.

4. Stay updated with evidence-based practices and guidelines: Keep yourself informed about current research, evidence-based practices, and clinical guidelines related to primary care and family practice nursing. Access resources provided by professional organizations, such as the American Association of Nurse Practitioners (AANP) or the American Academy of Family Physicians (AAFP).

5. Networking and professional involvement: Engage with professional organizations, such as the American Academy of Ambulatory Care Nursing (AAACN), the AANP, or the AAFP, to connect with other family practice nurses, access educational resources, and stay informed about emerging practices and career opportunities.

Remember that specific requirements and preferences may vary depending on the healthcare organization, geographical location, and level of experience desired for family practice nursing positions.

| Occupational Health Nursing |

Occupational health nursing is a specialized field that focuses on promoting and maintaining the health, safety, and well-being of workers in various industries. Occupational health nurses work in a range of settings, including workplaces, industrial facilities, government agencies, and healthcare organizations. They play a crucial role in assessing workplace hazards, implementing health and safety programs, providing employee education, managing workplace injuries, and facilitating return-to-work processes.

A Day in the Life

A typical day in the life of an occupational health nurse may involve:

1. Assessing and evaluating workplace environments to identify potential health and safety hazards, including physical, chemical, biological, ergonomic, and psychosocial factors.
2. Conducting pre-employment screenings, including medical history assessments and physical examinations, to ensure employees are fit to perform their job duties.
3. Developing and implementing health promotion and wellness programs, such as immunization campaigns, smoking cessation initiatives, and stress management workshops.
4. Providing education and training to employees on occupational health and safety topics, including proper use of personal protective equipment, safe work practices, and injury prevention.
5. Collaborating with management and human resources to develop policies and procedures that align with occupational health regulations and best practices.
6. Conducting health risk assessments and surveillance programs to monitor employee health and identify any occupational health concerns.
7. Managing workplace injuries and illnesses, including providing initial first aid, evaluating injuries, coordinating medical treatment, and facilitating workers' compensation processes.
8. Assisting in the development and implementation of return-to-work programs, including coordinating modified duty assignments and facilitating the rehabilitation process for injured employees.
9. Engaging in health promotion and injury prevention campaigns specific to the workplace, such as ergonomic assessments, hearing conservation programs, or chemical exposure monitoring.
10. Engaging in ongoing education and professional development to stay updated on the latest advancements in occupational health nursing, regulatory requirements, and evidence-based practices.

Degree(s) Required

To become an occupational health nurse, you need to earn a degree in nursing. The two common degree paths are an Associate Degree in Nursing (ADN) or a Bachelor of Science in Nursing (BSN). However, some employers may prefer or require a BSN for occupational health nursing positions due to the comprehensive knowledge and critical thinking skills gained.

Salary

$66,640 - $110,930

Specialty Certifications Available or Needed

Certification in occupational health nursing can demonstrate specialized knowledge and competence. The American Board for Occupational Health Nurses (ABOHN) offers the Certified Occupational Health Nurse (COHN) credential. Eligibility for the COHN certification typically requires a combination of education, clinical experience in occupational health nursing, and successful completion of an exam.

Job Requirements

Occupational health nursing requires a strong foundation in nursing practice, as well as additional knowledge and skills specific to workplace health and safety. Job requirements may include:

1. Proficiency in assessing workplace health hazards, including knowledge of occupational health regulations, hazard identification techniques, and risk assessment methods.

2. Understanding of common occupational health concerns, such as musculoskeletal injuries, chemical exposures, respiratory conditions, and stress-related disorders.

3. Familiarity with occupational health and safety standards, including knowledge of relevant regulations, best practices, and industry-specific guidelines.

4. Effective communication and education skills to provide comprehensive training and counseling to employees on occupational health and safety topics.

5. Collaboration with management, human resources, and occupational health professionals to develop and implement workplace health and safety programs and policies.

6. Proficiency in documentation and record-keeping, ensuring accurate and complete documentation of workplace assessments, employee health records, and injury reports.

7. Ability to adapt to a variety of work environments and industries,

understanding the specific hazards and risks associated with each.

8. Knowledge of workers' compensation processes, including managing workplace injuries, coordinating medical treatment, and facilitating the return-to-work process.

9. Understanding of legal and ethical considerations related to occupational health nursing, including privacy laws, worker's rights, and confidentiality requirements.

10. Ability to stay updated with current research, evidence-based practices, and regulatory requirements related to occupational health nursing.

Miscellaneous Information You Should Know

To enter the occupational health nursing specialty, you may consider the following:

1. Gain clinical experience in occupational health or related areas: Acquire experience in occupational health clinics, industrial facilities, or healthcare organizations with occupational health services to develop a foundation in workplace health assessments, injury management, and health promotion programs.

2. Pursue additional education or certifications in occupational health nursing: Consider attending workshops, seminars, or specialized training programs in occupational health nursing to enhance your knowledge and skills. These programs can provide education on workplace hazard assessments, regulatory requirements, and evidence-based practices in occupational health.

3. Stay updated with evidence-based practices: Keep yourself informed about current research, evidence-based practices, and regulatory requirements related to occupational health nursing. Access resources provided by professional organizations, such as the American Association of Occupational Health Nurses (AAOHN), to stay up-to-date with emerging practices and advancements in the field.

4. Networking and professional involvement: Engage with professional organizations and communities focused on occupational health nursing to connect with other occupational health nurses, access educational resources, and stay informed about career opportunities. Participate in conferences, webinars, or local chapter meetings to expand your knowledge and network with professionals in the field.

Remember that specific requirements and preferences may vary depending on the healthcare organization, geographical location, and industry in which you plan to practice occupational health nursing.

| Allergy and Immunology Nursing |

Allergy and Immunology Nursing is a specialized field of nursing that focuses on the care and management of patients with allergies, immune system disorders, and related conditions. Allergy and Immunology Nurses work closely with patients of all ages, providing education, conducting assessments, performing diagnostic tests, administering treatments, and managing ongoing care. They play a critical role in helping patients understand and manage their allergies, immunodeficiencies, and autoimmune disorders, as well as providing support and guidance in maintaining a healthy lifestyle.

A Day in the Life

A typical day in the life of an Allergy and Immunology Nurse may involve:

1. Patient Assessments: Conducting comprehensive assessments of patients to gather information about their medical history, allergy triggers, symptoms, and overall health. Assessments may include physical examinations, reviewing medical records, and administering allergy tests.

2. Allergy Testing: Administering and interpreting allergy tests such as skin prick tests, patch tests, or blood tests to identify specific allergens that trigger allergic reactions in patients.

3. Patient Education: Providing education to patients and their families about allergic conditions, including triggers, avoidance strategies, medication administration, and emergency management plans. Educating patients about immunodeficiency disorders, autoimmune conditions, and treatment options.

4. Treatment Administration: Administering medications such as allergy shots (immunotherapy), sublingual immunotherapy (SLIT), or biologic therapies as prescribed by the allergist or immunologist. Monitoring patients for adverse reactions and providing appropriate interventions.

5. Asthma Management: Assisting in the management of asthma in patients with allergic asthma. Educating patients on proper inhaler techniques, asthma action plans, and triggers avoidance.

6. Collaborative Care: Collaborating with allergists, immunologists, respiratory therapists, and other healthcare professionals to develop and implement individualized care plans for patients. Participating in interdisciplinary team meetings and contributing to the development of treatment protocols.

7. Documentation: Ensuring accurate and thorough documentation of patient assessments, interventions, treatments, and outcomes in medical records. Adhering to legal and ethical standards for documentation and

maintaining patient privacy and confidentiality.

8. Ongoing Patient Support: Providing ongoing support to patients with chronic allergies or immune disorders, including monitoring their progress, adjusting treatment plans as needed, and helping them manage their condition effectively. Assisting patients in accessing additional resources or referrals when necessary.

9. Community Education: Participating in community education initiatives to raise awareness about allergies, immunodeficiencies, and related conditions. Conducting public health campaigns, presenting educational sessions, or organizing support groups.

10. Continual Learning: Staying updated on current research, guidelines, and advancements in allergy and immunology nursing through professional development activities, attending conferences, and participating in specialty-specific workshops and seminars.

Degree(s) Required

To become an Allergy and Immunology Nurse, you need to earn a degree in nursing. The two common degree paths are an Associate Degree in Nursing (ADN) or a Bachelor of Science in Nursing (BSN). However, some employers may prefer or require a BSN due to its comprehensive curriculum and broader range of nursing skills.

Salary
$66,640 - $110,930

Specialty Certifications Available or Needed

Obtaining specialty certification in Allergy and Immunology Nursing can validate advanced knowledge and expertise in this field. The American Nurses Credentialing Center (ANCC) offers the Certified Allergy & Immunology Nurse (CAIN) certification, which demonstrates specialized knowledge and skills in caring for patients with allergies and immune disorders.

Job Requirements

Allergy and Immunology Nurses require specific knowledge and skills to provide effective care to patients with allergies, immunodeficiencies, and autoimmune conditions. Job requirements may include:

1. Knowledge of Allergies and Immunology: Proficiency in understanding the various types of allergies, immunodeficiencies, and autoimmune disorders, as well as their causes, symptoms, diagnostic tests, and treatment options.

2. Allergy Testing and Interpretation: Competence in administering and

interpreting allergy tests such as skin prick tests, patch tests, or blood tests. Understanding the significance of test results and using them to guide patient care.

3. Medication Administration: Familiarity with common medications used in allergy and immunology, including antihistamines, corticosteroids, immunosuppressants, and biologic therapies. Knowledge of proper administration techniques, potential side effects, and patient monitoring.

4. Asthma Management: Understanding the pathophysiology of asthma and proficiency in assisting patients with asthma management. Knowledge of different types of inhalers, spacers, and proper inhaler techniques.

5. Patient Education: Ability to provide patient and family education on allergic conditions, immune disorders, and treatment options. Clear communication skills to explain complex medical concepts in a way that patients can understand and apply in their daily lives.

6. Collaboration and Communication: Collaboration with allergists, immunologists, and other healthcare professionals to develop and implement comprehensive care plans. Effective communication and interdisciplinary teamwork are crucial.

7. Documentation: Ensuring accurate and thorough documentation of patient assessments, interventions, treatments, and outcomes in medical records. Adhering to legal and ethical standards for documentation.

8. Continuous Professional Development: Engaging in continuing education activities, attending conferences, and staying updated on current research and advancements in the field of allergy and immunology nursing.

Miscellaneous Information You Should Know

To enter the Allergy and Immunology Nursing specialty, you may consider the following:

1. Gain Clinical Experience: Seek opportunities to work in settings where you can gain exposure to patients with allergies, immunodeficiencies, or autoimmune disorders. This experience will provide a foundation for developing skills specific to this specialty.

2. Certification and Continuing Education: Pursue specialty certification as a Certified Allergy & Immunology Nurse (CAIN) through the American Nurses Credentialing Center (ANCC). Additionally, engage in continuing education activities and attend conferences or workshops focused on allergy and immunology nursing to expand your knowledge and stay updated on advancements in the field.

3. Networking and Professional Organizations: Connect with other Allergy and Immunology Nurses and join professional organizations such as the American Association of Allergy, Asthma & Immunology (AAAAI) or the Association of Asthma Educators (AAE). These organizations offer

resources, educational opportunities, and networking events specific to the field of allergy and immunology nursing.

4. Preceptorship and Mentorship: Seek opportunities to work with experienced Allergy and Immunology Nurses who can serve as mentors and provide guidance as you develop your skills in this specialty. Consider pursuing a preceptorship or mentorship program to enhance your learning experience.

5. Strong Patient Education Skills: Develop strong patient education skills to effectively educate and empower patients and their families to manage their allergies, immunodeficiencies, or autoimmune conditions. Adapt your communication style to meet the diverse needs of patients and ensure they understand their condition and treatment plan.

Remember that specific requirements and preferences may vary depending on the employer, healthcare facility, or allergy and immunology practice where you plan to work as an Allergy and Immunology Nurse.

| Forensic Nursing |

Forensic nursing is a specialized field that combines healthcare and the legal system. Forensic nurses provide care to individuals who have been affected by violence, trauma, or criminal activity. They play a crucial role in collecting evidence, providing support to victims, and collaborating with law enforcement and legal professionals. Forensic nurses work in a variety of settings, including hospitals, clinics, correctional facilities, and forensic laboratories.

A Day in the Life

A typical day in the life of a forensic nurse may involve:

1. Conducting assessments and examinations of patients who have experienced violence or trauma, including victims of sexual assault, domestic violence, child abuse, or elder abuse.
2. Collecting and preserving evidence, such as DNA samples, photographs, or injury documentation, using forensic techniques.
3. Providing compassionate and trauma-informed care to survivors, addressing their physical, emotional, and psychological needs.
4. Collaborating with law enforcement agencies, attorneys, and other members of the legal system to assist in investigations and legal proceedings.
5. Testifying as an expert witness in court regarding medical findings, evidence collection, and interpretation.
6. Educating healthcare professionals, law enforcement personnel, and the community about forensic nursing principles, violence prevention, and proper evidence handling.
7. Participating in multidisciplinary teams and case conferences to ensure comprehensive care for patients and coordination of services.
8. Documenting patient assessments, treatments, and evidence collection accurately and according to legal and professional standards.

Degree(s) Required

To become a forensic nurse, you need to earn a degree in nursing. The two common degree paths are an Associate Degree in Nursing (ADN) or a Bachelor of Science in Nursing (BSN). However, pursuing a BSN is increasingly preferred for forensic nursing positions due to the comprehensive knowledge and critical thinking skills gained. Additionally, specialized education or training in forensic nursing can enhance your expertise in this field.

Salary
$66,640 - $110,930

Specialty Certifications Available or Needed
Certification in forensic nursing can demonstrate specialized knowledge and competence. The International Association of Forensic Nurses (IAFN) offers the Sexual Assault Nurse Examiner (SANE) certification, which is specifically focused on caring for victims of sexual assault. The American Board of Nursing Specialties (ABNS) also recognizes forensic nursing as a specialty and offers certifications through various organizations. It is essential to research and consider the specific certification requirements and options available based on your area of interest within forensic nursing.

Job Requirements
Forensic nursing requires a strong foundation in clinical nursing skills, along with additional knowledge and skills specific to forensic practice. Job requirements may include:

1. Proficiency in conducting comprehensive patient assessments, including physical and psychological evaluations of victims of violence or trauma.

2. Knowledge of forensic principles, evidence collection techniques, and forensic laboratory procedures.

3. Competence in performing forensic examinations, such as sexual assault forensic exams or injury documentation.

4. Understanding of legal and ethical considerations related to forensic nursing practice, including confidentiality, informed consent, and mandatory reporting requirements.

5. Effective communication skills to interact with patients, families, law enforcement personnel, attorneys, and other members of the legal system.

6. Collaboration with multidisciplinary teams, including law enforcement, social workers, prosecutors, and victim advocates, to ensure coordinated care and justice for victims.

7. Skill in providing trauma-informed care, crisis intervention, and emotional support to individuals who have experienced violence or trauma.

8. Ability to navigate the legal system and provide expert witness testimony when necessary.

Miscellaneous Information You Should Know
To enter the forensic nursing specialty, you may consider the following:

1. Gain clinical experience in relevant areas: Acquire experience in emergency departments, trauma centers, or settings that provide care to

victims of violence or trauma. This experience will provide a foundation in assessing and managing patients who have experienced violence or trauma.

2. Pursue additional education or training in forensic nursing: Consider pursuing specialized education or training programs in forensic nursing. These programs can provide advanced knowledge and skills in evidence collection, forensic examination techniques, and legal considerations.

3. Develop strong communication and advocacy skills: Effective communication and advocacy are essential in forensic nursing. Enhance your ability to communicate sensitively and compassionately with survivors of violence or trauma. Learn how to advocate for patients' rights and collaborate with professionals in the legal system.

4. Gain knowledge of legal and ethical considerations: Familiarize yourself with the legal and ethical aspects of forensic nursing, including relevant laws, regulations, and standards of practice. Stay updated on changes in legislation and legal procedures that may impact forensic nursing practice.

5. Networking and professional involvement: Engage with professional organizations such as the International Association of Forensic Nurses (IAFN) to connect with other forensic nurses, access educational resources, and stay informed about emerging practices and career opportunities in forensic nursing.

Remember that specific requirements and preferences may vary depending on the healthcare organization, geographical location, and level of experience desired for forensic nursing positions. Additionally, some roles within forensic nursing, such as Sexual Assault Nurse Examiner (SANE) positions, may have additional requirements, such as completion of specialized training programs or clinical hours.

| Research Nursing |

Research nursing is a specialized field that focuses on the coordination and implementation of clinical research studies. Research nurses play a vital role in advancing healthcare by contributing to the development of new treatments, medications, and healthcare interventions. They collaborate with interdisciplinary teams, including researchers, physicians, pharmacists, and statisticians, to conduct research studies and ensure the safety and well-being of study participants. Research nurses can work in various settings, including academic institutions, hospitals, pharmaceutical companies, and research organizations.

A Day in the Life

A typical day in the life of a research nurse may involve:

1. Protocol Development: Collaborating with researchers and study teams to develop research protocols, including determining study objectives, participant eligibility criteria, data collection methods, and ethical considerations.

2. Participant Recruitment: Identifying and screening potential study participants, obtaining informed consent, and ensuring participants meet the eligibility criteria for enrollment in research studies.

3. Study Coordination: Overseeing the day-to-day operations of research studies, including scheduling study visits, coordinating study procedures, and managing study documents and records.

4. Data Collection and Management: Collecting and recording accurate and complete data from study participants, ensuring data integrity and adherence to research protocols. Managing data entry, data verification, and data quality control.

5. Participant Monitoring: Monitoring the safety and well-being of study participants, conducting assessments, and addressing any adverse events or concerns that may arise during the course of the study.

6. Compliance and Ethics: Ensuring compliance with ethical standards, regulations, and institutional review board (IRB) requirements for the protection of study participants' rights and safety.

7. Collaboration with the Research Team: Collaborating with researchers, statisticians, and other members of the research team to analyze and interpret research data, contribute to research publications, and disseminate research findings.

8. Education and Counseling: Providing education to study participants about the research study, its purpose, procedures, and potential risks or benefits. Offering counseling and support to address participants' questions

or concerns.

9. Documentation and Record-Keeping: Maintaining accurate and detailed documentation of study procedures, participant visits, and research data. Ensuring compliance with regulatory standards and healthcare policies.

10. Ongoing Education: Engaging in continuous learning and professional development to stay updated on research methodologies, ethical considerations, data management, and emerging trends in research nursing.

Degree(s) Required

To become a research nurse, you need to earn a degree in nursing. The two common degree paths are an Associate Degree in Nursing (ADN) or a Bachelor of Science in Nursing (BSN). However, some employers may prefer or require a BSN for research nursing positions due to the comprehensive knowledge and critical thinking skills gained. A BSN may also open up opportunities for research nursing roles with more responsibility and involvement in study design and data analysis.

Salary

$70,670 - $120,690

Specialty Certifications Available or Needed

Certification in research nursing can demonstrate specialized knowledge and competence. The Society of Clinical Research Associates (SoCRA) offers the Certified Clinical Research Professional (CCRP) credential. The Association of Clinical Research Professionals (ACRP) offers the Certified Clinical Research Coordinator (CCRC) and Certified Clinical Research Associate (CCRA) credentials. These certifications typically require a combination of education, clinical research experience, and successful completion of an exam.

Job Requirements

Research nursing requires a strong foundation in nursing practice, as well as additional knowledge and skills specific to clinical research. Job requirements may include:

1. Knowledge of research methodologies and study design, including the ability to understand and interpret research protocols.

2. Familiarity with research regulations and ethical considerations, including protection of human subjects, informed consent, and Institutional Review Board (IRB) requirements.

3. Proficiency in participant recruitment and screening, including

informed consent procedures and eligibility assessment.

4. Competence in data collection methods, including standardized assessments, surveys, and electronic data capture systems.

5. Understanding of Good Clinical Practice (GCP) guidelines, research documentation, and record-keeping practices to ensure compliance and data integrity.

6. Collaboration and communication skills to work effectively with interdisciplinary research teams, including researchers, statisticians, and pharmacists.

7. Attention to detail and data management skills to accurately collect, record, and manage research data.

8. Familiarity with research regulatory compliance, including reporting adverse events, monitoring study progress, and maintaining documentation.

9. Ability to provide education and counseling to research participants, including explaining study procedures, risks, and benefits.

10. Ability to stay updated with current research regulations, guidelines, and industry best practices in clinical research.

Miscellaneous Information You Should Know

To enter the research nursing specialty, you may consider the following:

1. Gain clinical experience in research settings: Seek opportunities to gain experience in research settings, such as academic institutions or hospitals conducting clinical trials. This experience will provide valuable exposure to research processes, regulatory compliance, and study coordination.

2. Pursue additional education or certifications in research nursing: Consider attending workshops, seminars, or specialized training programs in research nursing to enhance your knowledge and skills. These programs can provide education on research methodologies, data management, regulatory compliance, and ethical considerations.

3. Stay updated with current research practices: Stay informed about current research regulations, guidelines, and ethical considerations. Regularly access resources provided by professional organizations, such as the Society of Clinical Research Associates (SoCRA) and the Association of Clinical Research Professionals (ACRP), to stay up-to-date with emerging practices and advancements in the field.

4. Networking and professional involvement: Engage with professional organizations and communities focused on research nursing to connect with other research nurses, and access educational resources.

Remember that specific requirements and preferences may vary depending on the healthcare organization, research institution, geographical location, and level of experience desired for research nursing positions.

| Bariatric Nursing |

Bariatric Nursing is a specialized field of nursing that focuses on the care and management of patients who undergo bariatric surgery or have obesity-related health conditions. Bariatric Nurses work closely with patients to provide comprehensive pre-operative and post-operative care, including education, counseling, and ongoing support. They play a crucial role in helping patients achieve weight loss, improve their overall health, and prevent complications associated with obesity.

A Day in the Life

A typical day in the life of a Bariatric Nurse may involve:

1. Patient Assessments: Conducting comprehensive assessments of patients to gather information about their medical history, obesity-related health conditions, dietary habits, and overall health. Assessing patients for potential surgical risks and evaluating their readiness for bariatric surgery.

2. Pre-operative Education: Providing patients with detailed information about the bariatric surgery process, including the different surgical options, potential risks and benefits, dietary changes, and lifestyle modifications. Addressing any concerns or questions patients may have.

3. Collaborative Care: Collaborating with the bariatric surgical team, including surgeons, dietitians, psychologists, and other healthcare professionals, to develop individualized care plans for patients. Participating in interdisciplinary team meetings and contributing to the development of treatment protocols.

4. Post-operative Care: Monitoring patients closely after bariatric surgery to ensure proper healing, manage pain, and prevent complications. Educating patients on post-operative dietary guidelines, physical activity, medication management, and follow-up appointments.

5. Patient Support: Providing ongoing support and counseling to patients throughout their weight loss journey. Assisting patients in setting realistic goals, addressing emotional and psychological concerns, and developing healthy lifestyle habits.

6. Nutrition Counseling: Collaborating with dietitians to provide nutritional counseling and education to patients, including guidance on portion control, balanced diets, micronutrient supplementation, and long-term dietary changes.

7. Complication Management: Recognizing and managing potential complications related to bariatric surgery, such as wound infections, anastomotic leaks, nutrient deficiencies, or dumping syndrome. Monitoring patients for signs of complications and providing appropriate interventions or referrals.

8. Patient Advocacy: Serving as an advocate for patients by ensuring their rights, needs, and preferences are respected. Supporting patients in accessing resources, community support groups, and follow-up care.

9. Documentation: Ensuring accurate and thorough documentation of patient assessments, interventions, treatments, and outcomes in medical records. Adhering to legal and ethical standards for documentation and maintaining patient privacy and confidentiality.

10. Continual Learning: Staying updated on current research, guidelines, and advancements in bariatric nursing through professional development activities, attending conferences, and participating in specialty-specific workshops and seminars.

Degree(s) Required

To become a Bariatric Nurse, you need to earn a degree in nursing. The two common degree paths are an Associate Degree in Nursing (ADN) or a Bachelor of Science in Nursing (BSN). However, some employers may prefer or require a BSN due to its comprehensive curriculum and broader range of nursing skills.

Salary

$66,640 - $110,930

Specialty Certifications Available or Needed

Obtaining specialty certification in Bariatric Nursing can validate advanced knowledge and expertise in this field. The American Society for Metabolic and Bariatric Surgery (ASMBS) offers the Certified Bariatric Nurse (CBN) certification, which demonstrates specialized knowledge and skills in the care of bariatric surgery patients.

Job Requirements

Bariatric Nurses require specific knowledge and skills to provide effective care to patients undergoing bariatric surgery or managing obesity-related health conditions. Job requirements may include:

1. Knowledge of Bariatric Surgery: Proficiency in understanding different types of bariatric surgeries, their indications, potential risks and benefits, and expected outcomes. Familiarity with pre-operative evaluation criteria and post-operative management guidelines.

2. Nutrition and Dietetics: Understanding principles of nutrition, dietary counseling, and the specific dietary needs of bariatric surgery patients. Collaborating with dietitians to develop appropriate dietary plans and educate patients on nutritional requirements.

3. Patient Education and Counseling: Ability to provide patient and

family education on bariatric surgery procedures, dietary changes, lifestyle modifications, and long-term weight management. Skills in addressing patient concerns, providing emotional support, and promoting patient motivation and adherence to treatment plans.

4. Collaboration and Communication: Collaboration with the bariatric surgical team, including surgeons, dietitians, psychologists, and other healthcare professionals, to provide holistic care for bariatric patients. Effective communication and interdisciplinary teamwork are crucial.

5. Complication Management: Knowledge of potential post-operative complications, their signs and symptoms, and appropriate interventions. Skills in recognizing and managing complications related to wound healing, infections, nutritional deficiencies, or psychological issues.

6. Documentation: Ensuring accurate and thorough documentation of patient assessments, interventions, treatments, and outcomes in medical records. Adhering to legal and ethical standards for documentation.

7. Continuous Professional Development: Engaging in continuing education activities, attending conferences, and staying updated on current research and advancements in the field of bariatric nursing.

Miscellaneous Information You Should Know

To enter the Bariatric Nursing specialty, you may consider the following:

1. Gain Clinical Experience: Seek opportunities to work in settings that provide care for bariatric surgery patients, such as bariatric surgery centers, hospitals, or outpatient clinics. This experience will provide a foundation for developing skills specific to this specialty.

2. Certification and Continuing Education: Pursue specialty certification as a Certified Bariatric Nurse (CBN) through the American Society for Metabolic and Bariatric Surgery (ASMBS). Additionally, engage in continuing education activities and attend conferences or workshops focused on bariatric nursing to expand your knowledge and stay updated on advancements in the field.

3. Networking and Professional Organizations: Connect with other Bariatric Nurses and join professional organizations such as the American Society for Metabolic and Bariatric Surgery (ASMBS) or the Obesity Medicine Association (OMA). These organizations offer resources, educational opportunities, and networking events specific to the field of bariatric nursing.

4. Preceptorship and Mentorship: Seek opportunities to work with experienced Bariatric Nurses who can serve as mentors and provide guidance as you develop your skills in this specialty. Consider pursuing a preceptorship or mentorship program to enhance your learning experience.

5. Strong Patient Education Skills: Develop strong patient education

skills to effectively educate and empower patients and their families to manage their condition, adhere to dietary changes, and adopt a healthy lifestyle.

Remember that specific requirements and preferences may vary depending on the employer, healthcare facility, or bariatric practice where you plan to work as a Bariatric Nurse.

| Health Informatics Nursing |

Health Informatics Nursing combines the fields of nursing and information technology to improve healthcare outcomes through the use of data, technology, and informatics principles. Health Informatics Nurses play a critical role in managing, analyzing, and utilizing healthcare data to enhance patient care, streamline workflows, support clinical decision-making, and optimize healthcare systems and processes.

A Day in the Life

A typical day in the life of a Health Informatics Nurse may involve:

1. Data Management: Collecting, organizing, and managing healthcare data from various sources, including electronic health records (EHRs), health information systems, medical devices, and other healthcare technologies.

2. Data Analysis: Analyzing healthcare data to identify trends, patterns, and insights that can improve patient care, quality measures, and healthcare outcomes.

3. System Implementation and Optimization: Collaborating with interdisciplinary teams to implement and optimize electronic health record systems, clinical decision support tools, and other health information technologies.

4. Workflow Design: Assessing and redesigning clinical workflows to improve efficiency, patient safety, and data integrity within healthcare settings.

5. User Support and Training: Providing training and support to healthcare professionals on the use of health information technologies and ensuring compliance with privacy and security regulations.

6. Quality Improvement: Participating in quality improvement initiatives, such as developing and implementing evidence-based protocols and guidelines, and monitoring performance indicators.

7. Informatics Consultation: Serving as a subject matter expert in health informatics, collaborating with healthcare teams to develop informatics solutions that meet specific clinical and operational needs.

8. Project Management: Leading or participating in health informatics projects, such as system upgrades, integration of new technologies, or data migration initiatives.

9. Data Privacy and Security: Ensuring the confidentiality, integrity, and availability of healthcare data, and complying with privacy and security regulations, such as the Health Insurance Portability and Accountability Act (HIPAA).

10. Research and Innovation: Contributing to research studies and

staying abreast of emerging trends and technologies in health informatics to drive innovation and improve patient outcomes.

Degree(s) Required

To pursue a career in Health Informatics Nursing, a minimum of a Bachelor of Science in Nursing (BSN) degree is typically required. However, many positions may prefer or require a Master of Science in Nursing (MSN) or a graduate degree in Health Informatics, Nursing Informatics, or a related field. Advanced degrees provide a deeper understanding of informatics principles, data management, and healthcare technology.

Salary

$66,640 - $110,930

Specialty Certifications Available or Needed

Certifications can enhance your expertise in Health Informatics Nursing. Here are some certifications available:

1. Nursing Informatics Certification: The American Nurses Credentialing Center (ANCC) offers the Informatics Nursing Certification (RN-BC) for Registered Nurses interested in the field of nursing informatics.

2. Healthcare Information and Management Systems Society (HIMSS) Certifications: HIMSS offers various certifications, including the Certified Professional in Healthcare Information and Management Systems (CPHIMS) and the Certified Associate in Healthcare Information and Management Systems (CAHIMS), which validate expertise in health information technology and management.

3. Epic Certification: Epic Systems, a widely used electronic health record (EHR) system, offers certifications for healthcare professionals who specialize in implementing and using their software.

Specific certification requirements may vary, and it's important to research and identify certifications that align with your career goals and the specific systems or technologies you work with.

Job Requirements

To work in Health Informatics Nursing, consider the following job requirements:

1. Strong Background in Nursing: A solid foundation in nursing practice and understanding of healthcare workflows, patient care processes, and

clinical terminology are essential to effectively work with healthcare data and technology.

2. Knowledge of Health Information Systems: Familiarity with electronic health record (EHR) systems, health information exchange (HIE), clinical decision support systems, and other health information technologies used in healthcare settings.

3. Informatics Knowledge: Understanding of informatics principles, data management, data analysis, clinical terminology standards (e.g., SNOMED CT, LOINC), and health information exchange standards (e.g., HL7).

4. Technological Aptitude: Comfort and proficiency with technology, including computer skills, data analytics tools, and familiarity with data visualization and reporting tools.

5. Communication and Collaboration: Effective communication and collaboration skills to work with interdisciplinary teams, translate technical concepts to non-technical stakeholders, and facilitate change management.

6. Data Privacy and Security: Knowledge of privacy regulations, such as HIPAA, and the ability to apply security best practices to protect healthcare data.

7. Project Management: Basic project management skills to plan, coordinate, and execute health informatics initiatives, including system implementations and workflow redesigns.

8. Continuous Learning: Commitment to staying updated with evolving healthcare technologies, informatics standards, and regulations through professional development, certifications, and participation in relevant conferences or associations.

Miscellaneous Information You Should Know

To enter the field of Health Informatics Nursing, consider the following:

1. Gain Experience: Seek opportunities to gain experience in healthcare settings emphasizing health informatics, such as participating in informatics projects or working with electronic health records (EHRs) and health information systems.

2. Pursue Advanced Education: Consider pursuing a Master's degree or specialized training in Health Informatics, Nursing Informatics, or a related field to gain in-depth knowledge and skills in health data management, health technology, and informatics principles.

3. Networking and Professional Engagement: Join professional organizations related to health informatics and nursing informatics, such as the American Medical Informatics Association (AMIA) and the Healthcare Information and Management Systems Society (HIMSS).

Working in Health Informatics Nursing allows you to combine your nursing expertise with technology and data management skills to contribute to improving healthcare outcomes and the efficient delivery of care.

| Nurse Educator |

Nurse Educators are registered nurses who specialize in teaching and educating aspiring nurses, current nursing students, and healthcare professionals. They play a critical role in preparing the next generation of nurses and facilitating the ongoing professional development of practicing nurses. Nurse Educators work in academic institutions, hospitals, healthcare organizations, and clinical settings to impart knowledge, skills, and competencies necessary for effective nursing practice.

A Day in the Life

A typical day in the life of a Nurse Educator may involve:

1. Curriculum Development: Designing, developing, and revising nursing curricula, course materials, and educational resources to ensure they align with current healthcare standards, evidence-based practices, and regulatory requirements.

2. Classroom Instruction: Conducting lectures, leading discussions, and facilitating interactive learning experiences to educate nursing students on various nursing concepts, theories, and clinical skills.

3. Clinical Training: Overseeing and coordinating clinical experiences and simulations for nursing students, providing guidance, feedback, and supervision during hands-on patient care activities.

4. Assessments and Evaluations: Developing and administering assessments, examinations, and evaluations to measure students' understanding and progress in the nursing program.

5. Mentorship and Guidance: Providing mentorship, guidance, and academic advising to nursing students, supporting their professional and personal development.

6. Faculty Collaboration: Collaborating with other faculty members, nursing program directors, and healthcare professionals to ensure the integration of current evidence-based practice and emerging trends into the nursing curriculum.

7. Professional Development: Engaging in continuous professional development activities, such as attending conferences, workshops, and seminars, to stay updated with the latest advancements in nursing education and teaching methodologies.

8. Research and Scholarship: Conducting nursing research, publishing scholarly articles, and contributing to the advancement of nursing knowledge and evidence-based practice.

9. Program Evaluation: Participating in the evaluation and accreditation processes of nursing programs, ensuring compliance with regulatory and quality standards.

10. Clinical Practice: Maintaining clinical competence by engaging in periodic clinical practice or maintaining a part-time clinical role to stay connected with current healthcare practices.

Degree(s) Required

To pursue a career as a Nurse Educator, a minimum of a Master of Science in Nursing (MSN) degree is typically required. Some positions or institutions may prefer or require a Doctor of Nursing Practice (DNP) or a Ph.D. in Nursing Education. It is essential to have a strong foundation in nursing practice and knowledge of advanced nursing concepts and theories.

Salary

$68,910 - $113,410

Specialty Certifications Available or Needed

While not mandatory, obtaining a certification in nursing education can demonstrate expertise and commitment to the field. The National League for Nursing (NLN) offers the Certified Nurse Educator (CNE) certification, which recognizes nurse educators who meet the eligibility criteria and pass a comprehensive examination.

Job Requirements

To work as a Nurse Educator, consider the following job requirements:

1. Nursing Experience: Prior clinical experience as a registered nurse is typically required to establish credibility and bring real-world examples into the teaching and mentoring role.
2. Teaching Skills: Proficiency in instructional methodologies, curriculum design, and educational technology to effectively engage students and facilitate their learning.
3. Communication and Interpersonal Skills: Excellent verbal and written communication skills to convey complex nursing concepts, provide feedback, and collaborate with students, faculty, and healthcare professionals.
4. Leadership Abilities: Strong leadership and organizational skills to manage the educational environment, coordinate student experiences, and foster a positive learning atmosphere.
5. Knowledge of Teaching Strategies: Familiarity with a variety of teaching strategies, such as active learning, problem-based learning, and simulation, to enhance student engagement and promote critical thinking.
6. Research and Scholarship: An understanding of nursing research principles, evidence-based practice, and the ability to integrate research findings into the teaching and learning process.

7. Professional Development: A commitment to ongoing professional development, staying updated with current nursing practice, educational trends, and teaching methodologies.

8. Collaboration: Ability to collaborate effectively with interdisciplinary healthcare teams, clinical partners, and community organizations to enhance nursing education and clinical experiences.

9. Regulatory and Accreditation Knowledge: Familiarity with nursing education regulations, accreditation requirements, and quality assurance processes to ensure compliance and maintain program accreditation.

Miscellaneous Information You Should Know

To enter the field of Nurse Educator, consider the following:

1. Advanced Education: Pursuing a master's or doctoral degree in nursing education or a related field can provide the necessary knowledge and skills to excel in this specialty.

2. Teaching Experience: Seek opportunities to gain teaching experience, such as serving as a clinical instructor or adjunct faculty member, to develop and demonstrate teaching capabilities.

3. Networking and Collaboration: Engage with other nurse educators, attend educational conferences, and join professional organizations such as the National League for Nursing (NLN) or the American Association of Colleges of Nursing (AACN) to network, share best practices, and access resources.

4. Continuing Education: Participate in continuing education programs, workshops, or online courses specifically designed for nurse educators to enhance teaching skills and stay updated with the evolving field of nursing education.

5. Publish and Present: Contribute to the field of nursing education by publishing scholarly articles, presenting at conferences, and sharing innovative teaching strategies or research findings.

Becoming a Nurse Educator allows nurses to make a significant impact on the future of nursing by shaping the knowledge, skills, and professionalism of future nurses. It offers opportunities to inspire and empower the next generation of healthcare professionals while contributing to the advancement of nursing education and practice.

| Managed Care Nursing |

Managed care nursing is a specialized field that focuses on coordinating and managing healthcare services for individuals enrolled in managed care plans. Managed care nurses work in various settings, including health insurance companies, health maintenance organizations (HMOs), or accountable care organizations (ACOs). They play a crucial role in assessing, planning, and coordinating healthcare services to ensure cost-effective and quality care for patients while promoting preventive measures and disease management.

A Day in the Life

A typical day in the life of a managed care nurse may involve:

1. Assessing and reviewing patient healthcare needs, medical records, and treatment plans to determine appropriate care and utilization of healthcare services.

2. Collaborating with healthcare providers, including physicians, specialists, and allied healthcare professionals, to coordinate patient care, streamline services, and ensure adherence to evidence-based guidelines.

3. Conducting utilization reviews to evaluate the medical necessity, appropriateness, and cost-effectiveness of medical procedures, hospital admissions, or other healthcare services.

4. Educating patients and their families on managed care plans, benefits, coverage limitations, and preventive measures to promote wellness and optimal health outcomes.

5. Developing care management plans, including identifying resources, coordinating referrals, and monitoring the progress of patients' healthcare goals.

6. Assisting with case management activities, such as coordinating care transitions, facilitating communication between providers, and advocating for patients' healthcare needs.

7. Analyzing healthcare data and outcomes to identify trends, patterns, and opportunities for quality improvement or cost containment.

8. Collaborating with the interdisciplinary team, including pharmacists, social workers, and healthcare administrators, to ensure coordinated care delivery and address patients' healthcare needs comprehensively.

9. Providing health education and counseling to patients, promoting self-care management, medication adherence, and lifestyle modifications.

10. Engaging in ongoing education and professional development to stay updated on the latest advancements in managed care, healthcare policies, and healthcare delivery models.

Degree(s) Required

To become a managed care nurse, you need to earn a degree in nursing. The two common degree paths are an Associate Degree in Nursing (ADN) or a Bachelor of Science in Nursing (BSN). However, some employers may prefer or require a BSN for managed care nursing positions due to the comprehensive knowledge and critical thinking skills gained.

Salary
$65,000 - $107,500

Specialty Certifications Available or Needed
While there isn't a specific certification dedicated solely to managed care nursing, certifications in case management or healthcare quality can demonstrate specialized knowledge and competence in these areas. The Commission for Case Manager Certification (CCMC) offers the Certified Case Manager (CCM) credential, which can be beneficial for managed care nurses involved in case management roles. Additionally, the National Association for Healthcare Quality (NAHQ) offers the Certified Professional in Healthcare Quality (CPHQ) credential, which focuses on quality improvement and patient safety.

Job Requirements
Managed care nursing requires a strong foundation in nursing practice, as well as additional knowledge and skills related to care coordination, utilization management, and healthcare policies. Job requirements may include:

1. Proficiency in assessing patient healthcare needs, reviewing medical records, and applying evidence-based guidelines to determine appropriate care and utilization of healthcare services.

2. Knowledge of managed care plans, health insurance policies, coverage limitations, and healthcare reimbursement mechanisms.

3. Understanding of healthcare utilization management processes, including conducting utilization reviews, managing referrals, and ensuring cost-effective care delivery.

4. Competence in case management principles, including developing care management plans, coordinating care transitions, and collaborating with healthcare providers to achieve patients' healthcare goals.

5. Familiarity with healthcare quality improvement methodologies and techniques to analyze healthcare data, identify trends, and implement quality improvement initiatives.

6. Effective communication and interpersonal skills to engage with patients, healthcare providers, and other stakeholders in a collaborative and patient-centered manner.

7. Collaboration with the interdisciplinary team, including physicians, specialists, pharmacists, and social workers, to ensure coordinated care delivery and promote positive health outcomes.

8. Proficiency in documentation and record-keeping, ensuring accurate and complete documentation of patient assessments, care plans, interventions, and outcomes.

Miscellaneous Information You Should Know

To enter the managed care nursing specialty, you may consider the following:

1. Gain clinical experience in relevant areas: Acquire experience in various healthcare settings, such as hospitals, clinics, or care management departments, to develop a solid foundation in nursing practice and patient care coordination.

2. Develop knowledge in managed care principles: Familiarize yourself with managed care concepts, health insurance policies, utilization management, and healthcare delivery models. Understand the roles and responsibilities of managed care nurses within different healthcare organizations.

3. Pursue additional education or certifications in case management or healthcare quality: Consider attending workshops, seminars, or specialized training programs in case management or healthcare quality to enhance your knowledge and skills. These programs can provide education on care coordination, utilization management, healthcare policies, and quality improvement methodologies.

4. Stay updated with industry changes and healthcare policies: Keep yourself informed about current healthcare policies, regulations, and advancements in managed care. Access resources provided by professional organizations, industry publications, and healthcare policy organizations to stay up-to-date with emerging practices and advancements in the field.

5. Networking and professional involvement: Engage with professional organizations and communities focused on managed care or care management to connect with other managed care nurses, access educational resources, and stay informed about career opportunities. Participate in conferences, webinars, or local chapter meetings to expand your knowledge and network with professionals in the field.

Remember that specific requirements and preferences may vary depending on the healthcare organization, geographical location, and level of experience desired for managed care nursing positions.

| Substance Abuse Nursing |

Substance Abuse Nursing, also known as Addiction Nursing or Chemical Dependency Nursing, is a specialized field of nursing that focuses on the care and treatment of individuals with substance abuse and addiction disorders. Substance Abuse Nurses play a crucial role in assessing, managing, and supporting patients through various stages of addiction, withdrawal, recovery, and relapse prevention. They work in a variety of settings, including detoxification centers, rehabilitation facilities, outpatient clinics, correctional facilities, and community health organizations.

A Day in the Life

A typical day in the life of a Substance Abuse Nurse may involve:

1. Assessment and Screening: Conducting comprehensive assessments and screenings to evaluate patients' substance abuse history, physical and mental health status, social circumstances, and treatment needs.

2. Care Planning: Collaborating with the interdisciplinary team, including physicians, counselors, and social workers, to develop individualized care plans and treatment goals for patients.

3. Medication Management: Administering medications, such as opioid agonists or antagonist medications, to assist with detoxification, manage withdrawal symptoms, or support medication-assisted treatment (MAT) programs.

4. Monitoring and Support: Monitoring patients for signs of withdrawal, managing withdrawal symptoms, and providing supportive care throughout the detoxification process.

5. Counseling and Education: Providing counseling and education to patients and their families regarding the effects of substance abuse, the process of recovery, relapse prevention strategies, and the importance of ongoing support systems.

6. Group Therapy: Facilitating or participating in group therapy sessions to promote peer support, share experiences, and foster a sense of community among patients.

7. Health Promotion: Promoting overall health and well-being by addressing co-occurring physical and mental health conditions, educating patients about harm reduction practices, and providing information on preventive health measures.

8. Case Management: Coordinating care and referrals for patients, including arranging follow-up appointments, connecting patients with community resources, and advocating for their needs within the healthcare system.

9. Documentation and Record-Keeping: Maintaining accurate and

detailed documentation of assessments, care plans, interventions, progress notes, and treatment outcomes, while adhering to legal and ethical standards.

10. Collaborative Care: Collaborating with other healthcare professionals, such as psychiatrists, psychologists, social workers, and addiction counselors, to provide comprehensive and integrated care for patients with substance abuse disorders.

Degree(s) Required

To become a Substance Abuse Nurse, you need to earn a degree in nursing. The two common degree paths are an Associate Degree in Nursing (ADN) or a Bachelor of Science in Nursing (BSN). However, some employers or substance abuse treatment centers may prefer or require a BSN due to the comprehensive knowledge and critical thinking skills gained.

Salary

$66,640 - $110,930

Specialty Certifications Available or Needed

Certification in Substance Abuse Nursing can demonstrate specialized knowledge and competence in this field. The International Nurses Society on Addictions (IntNSA) offers the Certified Addictions Registered Nurse (CARN) certification, which requires meeting specific education and practice requirements and passing an examination.

Job Requirements

Substance Abuse Nurses require specific knowledge and skills to effectively care for individuals with substance abuse disorders. Job requirements may include:

1. In-depth understanding of substance abuse disorders, including the physiological, psychological, and social aspects of addiction.

2. Knowledge of evidence-based practices for the treatment of substance abuse, including detoxification protocols, medication-assisted treatment (MAT), cognitive-behavioral therapies, motivational interviewing, and relapse prevention strategies.

3. Competence in assessing and managing withdrawal symptoms, recognizing signs of substance intoxication or overdose, and implementing appropriate interventions.

4. Proficiency in administering and monitoring medications commonly used in substance abuse treatment, such as opioid agonists (e.g., methadone, buprenorphine) or antagonist medications (e.g., naloxone).

5. Familiarity with community resources, support groups, and referral networks for ongoing care and recovery.

6. Excellent communication and counseling skills to build rapport with patients, provide education, and support behavior change.

7. Cultural sensitivity and awareness to address the unique needs and challenges faced by individuals from diverse backgrounds.

8. Non-judgmental and empathetic approach to foster a therapeutic alliance and establish a safe and supportive environment for patients.

9. Documentation and record-keeping skills to maintain accurate and confidential patient records, including assessments, treatment plans, progress notes, and discharge summaries.

10. Commitment to self-care and professional boundaries, as working in substance abuse nursing can be emotionally demanding. Awareness of personal biases and the ability to practice without prejudice or stigmatization is crucial.

Miscellaneous Information You Should Know

To enter the Substance Abuse Nursing specialty, you may consider the following:

1. Gain experience or pursue education in addiction nursing: Seek opportunities to work in addiction treatment settings, such as detoxification centers, rehabilitation facilities, or outpatient clinics, to gain hands-on experience in caring for individuals with substance abuse disorders. Additionally, pursue continuing education courses or workshops focused on addiction nursing to enhance your knowledge and skills in this specialty.

2. Engage in professional development and networking: Join professional organizations, such as the International Nurses Society on Addictions (IntNSA), to access resources, attend conferences, and connect with other professionals in the field of substance abuse nursing. Engaging in continuing education and networking opportunities can help you stay updated on best practices, research advancements, and emerging trends in addiction nursing.

3. Obtain additional certifications or credentials: Consider pursuing certifications or credentials related to addiction counseling or treatment, such as becoming a Certified Addiction Counselor (CAC) or Certified Alcohol and Drug Counselor (CADC).

Remember that specific requirements and preferences may vary depending on the employer, substance abuse treatment center, or region where you plan to practice as a Substance Abuse Nurse.

| Telephone Triage Nursing |

Telephone Triage Nursing is a specialized field of nursing that focuses on providing remote healthcare advice, assessment, and guidance to patients over the phone. Telephone Triage Nurses use their clinical expertise, critical thinking skills, and nursing knowledge to assess patients' symptoms, provide appropriate recommendations, and determine the level of care required. They work in various healthcare settings, such as telehealth call centers, nurse advice lines, and medical clinics, to assist patients in making informed decisions about their healthcare needs.

A Day in the Life

A typical day in the life of a Telephone Triage Nurse may involve:

1. Receiving Calls: Answering incoming calls from patients seeking medical advice or guidance. Gathering relevant information about the patient's symptoms, medical history, and current condition through effective questioning and active listening.

2. Assessing Patient Symptoms: Using clinical knowledge and assessment skills to evaluate the severity and urgency of the patient's symptoms. Applying evidence-based protocols or guidelines to determine the appropriate course of action.

3. Providing Medical Advice: Offering appropriate advice, education, and self-care instructions to patients based on their symptoms, medical history, and available resources. Recommending over-the-counter medications, home remedies, or when necessary, advising patients to seek further medical attention.

4. Referring to Healthcare Providers: Identifying situations that require immediate medical attention or follow-up care and referring patients to the appropriate healthcare providers or facilities. Coordinating appointments, if necessary, and ensuring seamless transitions of care.

5. Documenting Calls: Accurately documenting all relevant information from patient calls, including symptoms, assessments, recommendations, and referrals, following established protocols and documentation guidelines.

6. Collaborating with Healthcare Team: Communicating and collaborating with physicians, nurses, and other healthcare professionals to seek guidance, clarify concerns, or provide follow-up information as needed.

7. Patient Education: Providing patient education on preventive measures, managing chronic conditions, recognizing red flags, and promoting overall health and wellness.

8. Adhering to Protocols and Guidelines: Following established

protocols, triage algorithms, and evidence-based guidelines to ensure consistent and safe patient care.

9. Ensuring Confidentiality: Respecting patient privacy and adhering to strict confidentiality protocols when handling patient information over the phone.

10. Continuing Education: Engaging in ongoing professional development activities to stay updated on current healthcare practices, evidence-based guidelines, and emerging trends in telephone triage nursing.

Degree(s) Required

To become a Telephone Triage Nurse, you need to earn a degree in nursing. The two common degree paths are an Associate Degree in Nursing (ADN) or a Bachelor of Science in Nursing (BSN). However, some employers or telehealth call centers may prefer or require a BSN due to the comprehensive knowledge and critical thinking skills gained.

Salary

$66,640 - $110,930

Specialty Certifications Available or Needed

While not required, obtaining certification in Telephone Triage Nursing can demonstrate specialized knowledge and competence in this field. The American Academy of Ambulatory Care Nursing (AAACN) offers the Telephone Nursing Practice (TNP) certification, which validates the skills and knowledge necessary for telephone triage nursing.

Job Requirements

Telephone Triage Nurses require specific knowledge and skills to effectively assess and provide remote healthcare advice. Job requirements may include:

1. Strong Clinical Knowledge: Possessing a solid foundation of general nursing knowledge and understanding of common medical conditions, symptoms, and treatment options.

2. Excellent Communication Skills: Demonstrating effective verbal and written communication skills to interact with patients, gather information, and provide clear and concise instructions over the phone.

3. Critical Thinking and Decision-Making Skills: Applying critical thinking skills to assess patient symptoms, recognize potential emergencies, and make accurate clinical decisions based on available information.

4. Empathy and Compassion: Displaying empathy and compassion while providing care remotely to ensure patients feel heard, supported, and understood.

5. Ability to Work Independently: Being able to work autonomously, make sound decisions, and prioritize tasks in a fast-paced environment without direct supervision.

6. Technological Competence: Demonstrating proficiency in using telecommunication systems, electronic health records (EHRs), and computer software to document calls and access patient information.

7. Flexibility and Adaptability: Adapting to changing patient needs, varying call volumes, and evolving healthcare protocols and guidelines.

8. Time Management and Organizational Skills: Efficiently managing multiple calls, documenting information accurately, and adhering to established call handling times.

9. Multicultural Awareness: Recognizing and respecting cultural, linguistic, and diverse healthcare needs to provide patient-centered care to a wide range of populations.

10. Compliance and Legal Considerations: Understanding and adhering to legal and ethical standards, confidentiality regulations (such as HIPAA), and organizational policies related to telephone triage nursing.

Miscellaneous Information You Should Know

To enter the Telephone Triage Nursing specialty, you may consider the following:

1. Gain clinical experience: Acquire experience in a clinical setting, such as medical-surgical, emergency department, or ambulatory care, to develop a solid foundation in general nursing knowledge and clinical assessment skills.

2. Develop communication skills: Focus on improving communication skills, including active listening, effective questioning, and providing clear and concise instructions. These skills are crucial when interacting with patients remotely.

3. Seek telehealth training: Explore opportunities for telehealth training or certifications to gain expertise in remote patient care and familiarize yourself with telecommunication technologies and software commonly used in telephone triage nursing.

4. Stay updated on guidelines and protocols: Stay informed about evidence-based guidelines, protocols, and triage algorithms specific to telephone triage nursing.

5. Pursue certification in Telephone Triage Nursing, such as the Telephone Nursing Practice (TNP) certification offered by the American Academy of Ambulatory Care Nursing (AAACN), to validate your specialized knowledge and skills.

Remember that specific requirements may vary depending on the employer, telehealth call center, or region where you plan to practice as a Telephone Triage Nurse.

| Bioethics Nursing |

Bioethics Nursing is a specialized field of nursing that focuses on the ethical aspects of healthcare and the moral dilemmas that arise in patient care. Bioethics Nurses work in collaboration with patients, families, and interdisciplinary teams to navigate complex ethical issues, make informed decisions, and ensure that healthcare practices align with ethical principles and legal standards. They provide ethical consultation, support, and advocacy to promote patient autonomy, justice, and beneficence.

A Day in the Life
A typical day in the life of a Bioethics Nurse may involve:

1. Ethical Consultation: Participating in ethical consultations with healthcare providers, patients, and families to address ethical concerns and dilemmas. Collaborating with ethics committees or consult services to analyze ethical issues and provide guidance on ethical decision-making.

2. Patient Advocacy: Advocating for patients' rights, autonomy, and well-being in the face of complex medical decisions. Assisting patients and families in understanding their options, providing information on risks and benefits, and facilitating discussions on goals of care and treatment options.

3. Education and Training: Providing education and training on ethical principles, policies, and guidelines to healthcare professionals, patients, and families. Promoting ethical awareness and competence among the healthcare team.

4. Policy and Procedure Development: Contributing to the development and review of institutional policies, protocols, and guidelines related to ethical issues in healthcare. Ensuring that policies align with legal requirements and ethical standards.

5. Ethics Committee Participation: Serving as an active member of an ethics committee or consult service, attending meetings, reviewing cases, and offering recommendations for resolving ethical dilemmas. Collaborating with interdisciplinary team members to reach consensus on ethical decisions.

6. Research and Scholarship: Engaging in research and scholarship activities related to bioethics. Participating in ethical research practices, contributing to bioethical literature, and presenting findings at conferences or other educational forums.

7. Ethical Decision-Making Support: Assisting healthcare providers, patients, and families in navigating ethical decision-making processes. Providing a framework for ethical analysis, facilitating communication and dialogue, and helping individuals explore and understand different perspectives.

8. Policy Advocacy: Engaging in advocacy efforts to promote ethical practices and policies at the institutional, community, or legislative levels. Participating in discussions and initiatives related to healthcare ethics, patient rights, and ethical guidelines.

9. Confidentiality and Privacy: Respecting patient confidentiality and privacy while engaging in ethical discussions and consultations. Adhering to ethical principles and legal requirements for privacy and informed consent.

10. Continuing Education: Engaging in ongoing professional development and continuing education activities related to bioethics. Staying updated on current ethical debates, legal regulations, and advancements in the field.

Degree(s) Required

To become a Bioethics Nurse, you need to have a Bachelor of Science in Nursing (BSN) degree. Some institutions or organizations may prefer or require a Master's degree in Bioethics, Nursing Ethics, or a related field.

Salary

$65,430 - $116,790

Specialty Certifications Available or Needed

There are several specialty certifications available in the field of bioethics. While not specific to nursing, they can enhance your knowledge and credibility as a Bioethics Nurse. Some recognized certifications include:

1. Certified Clinical Ethicist (CCE): Offered by the American Society for Bioethics and Humanities (ASBH), this certification demonstrates expertise in clinical ethics consultation and ethical decision-making.

2. Certified Healthcare Ethics Consultant (CHEC): Offered by the Healthcare Ethics Consultants Certification Board (HECCB), this certification validates skills in ethical consultation, policy development, and education in healthcare settings.

Obtaining these certifications can enhance your competence and demonstrate your commitment to the field of bioethics.

Job Requirements

Bioethics Nurses require specific knowledge and skills to navigate complex ethical issues in healthcare. Job requirements may include:

1. Ethical Competence: Strong understanding of ethical principles, theories, and frameworks relevant to healthcare. Ability to apply ethical principles in clinical practice, policy development, and decision-making.

2. Communication and Collaboration: Excellent communication skills to engage in ethical discussions and consultations with healthcare professionals, patients, and families. Ability to collaborate effectively with interdisciplinary teams and respect diverse perspectives.

3. Critical Thinking: Strong analytical and critical thinking skills to assess complex ethical dilemmas, identify relevant ethical principles, and apply ethical frameworks in decision-making.

4. Knowledge of Legal and Regulatory Frameworks: Familiarity with relevant laws, regulations, and professional guidelines that inform ethical practices in healthcare, such as informed consent, patient autonomy, confidentiality, and end-of-life care.

5. Emotional Intelligence: Sensitivity to the emotional and psychological aspects of ethical decision-making and the ability to provide support and empathy to patients, families, and healthcare providers during difficult ethical discussions.

6. Research and Ethics Review: Understanding of research ethics and the ability to contribute to research protocols, informed consent processes, and ethical review boards.

7. Continuous Professional Development: Engaging in ongoing professional development activities, attending bioethics conferences, and staying updated on current ethical debates, policies, and advancements in the field.

Miscellaneous Information You Should Know

To enter the Bioethics Nursing specialty, you may consider the following:

1. Gain Clinical Experience: Develop a strong foundation in clinical nursing practice before pursuing a career in bioethics nursing. Acquire experience in diverse healthcare settings to gain exposure to various ethical dilemmas and decision-making processes.

2. Additional Education: Consider pursuing additional education, such as a Master's degree or certificate program in Bioethics or Nursing Ethics. This specialized education will provide you with a deeper understanding of ethical theory, principles, and practices.

3. Ethics Committees and Consultation Services: Seek opportunities to join ethics committees or participate in ethics consultation services within healthcare institutions. This involvement will allow you to gain practical experience in bioethics and contribute to ethical decision-making processes.

4. Professional Organizations: Join professional organizations such as the American Society for Bioethics and Humanities (ASBH) or other local and national bioethics organizations. These organizations offer resources, networking opportunities, and educational events related to bioethics.

5. Networking and Mentorship: Connect with experienced Bioethics Nurses or professionals in the field of bioethics. Networking and mentorship can provide valuable guidance, career advice, and opportunities for collaboration.

Remember that specific requirements and preferences may vary depending on the employer, healthcare institution, or organization where you plan to work as a Bioethics Nurse.

| Diabetes Education Nursing |

Diabetes Educator Nursing is a specialized field that focuses on providing education, support, and guidance to individuals with diabetes. Diabetes Educator Nurses work closely with patients to help them understand their condition, manage their diabetes effectively, and make lifestyle changes to improve their overall health. They play a crucial role in empowering patients to take control of their diabetes through education, self-care practices, and medication management.

A Day in the Life

A typical day in the life of a Diabetes Educator Nurse may involve:

1. Patient Assessment: Conducting comprehensive assessments of patients with diabetes, including reviewing medical histories, evaluating blood glucose levels, and assessing patients' understanding of diabetes management.

2. Education and Counseling: Providing individualized education and counseling sessions to patients to enhance their knowledge of diabetes, including topics such as blood glucose monitoring, medication management, dietary adjustments, physical activity, and lifestyle modifications.

3. Treatment Planning: Collaborating with patients to develop personalized diabetes management plans that align with their lifestyle, preferences, and specific needs.

4. Group Education: Conducting group education sessions to educate patients about diabetes prevention, management, and complications, and fostering peer support and sharing of experiences.

5. Self-Care Training: Teaching patients how to administer insulin, use glucose monitoring devices, and manage hypoglycemic and hyperglycemic episodes.

6. Medication Management: Assisting patients in understanding their prescribed medications, including insulin therapy, oral antidiabetic medications, and potential side effects.

7. Nutritional Guidance: Providing guidance on healthy eating habits, meal planning, carbohydrate counting, and portion control to help patients achieve glycemic control.

8. Exercise and Physical Activity: Educating patients on the benefits of regular physical activity and guiding them in developing exercise routines that suit their abilities and medical conditions.

9. Emotional Support: Addressing the emotional and psychological aspects of living with diabetes, such as stress management, coping strategies, and fostering resilience.

10. Continuous Monitoring: Monitoring patients' progress in managing their diabetes, tracking blood glucose levels, and evaluating the effectiveness of interventions.

11. Collaboration with Healthcare Team: Collaborating with other healthcare professionals, including physicians, dietitians, pharmacists, and diabetes specialists, to provide comprehensive and coordinated care to patients.

12. Documentation and Reporting: Maintaining accurate and up-to-date patient records, documenting assessments, education sessions, and progress made.

13. Research and Professional Development: Staying updated on the latest research, advancements, and best practices in diabetes management through continuous education, attending conferences, and engaging in professional development activities.

Degree(s) Required

To become a Diabetes Educator Nurse, you need to have a degree in nursing. The two common degree paths are an Associate Degree in Nursing (ADN) or a Bachelor of Science in Nursing (BSN). However, some employers may prefer or require a BSN due to the specialized nature of the role. Additionally, obtaining a Master of Science in Nursing (MSN) with a specialization in diabetes management can provide advanced knowledge and opportunities for leadership in the field.

Salary

$63,790 - $106,820

Specialty Certifications Available or Needed

Obtaining a specialty certification in diabetes education can showcase your expertise and commitment to this nursing specialty. The recognized certification for Diabetes Educator Nurses is:

1. Certified Diabetes Educator (CDE): Offered by the National Certification Board for Diabetes Educators (NCBDE), the CDE certification validates your knowledge and skills in diabetes management and education. It requires a combination of clinical experience in diabetes education and passing a comprehensive exam.

Having the CDE certification demonstrates your competency in providing evidence-based diabetes education, promoting self-care practices, and helping patients achieve optimal diabetes control.

Job Requirements

To work as a Diabetes Educator Nurse, consider the following job requirements:

1. Clinical Competence: Proficiency in diabetes management, including knowledge of various types of diabetes, medications, insulin administration, blood glucose monitoring, and complications associated with the disease.
2. Diabetes Education Expertise: Expertise in providing patient-centered diabetes education and counseling, including developing personalized diabetes management plans and empowering patients to make informed decisions regarding their health.
3. Communication and Teaching Skills: Excellent communication and teaching skills to effectively educate and support patients in understanding their condition, self-care practices, and behavior modifications.
4. Collaboration and Interdisciplinary Approach: Ability to work collaboratively with other healthcare professionals and community resources to provide comprehensive diabetes care.
5. Cultural Competence: Demonstrating cultural competence and sensitivity to address the diverse needs, beliefs, and values of individuals with diabetes from different cultural backgrounds.
6. Continuous Learning: Staying updated on the latest advancements, research, and best practices in diabetes management through ongoing education and professional development.
7. Emotional Intelligence: Possessing empathy, active listening skills, and the ability to establish rapport with patients, providing emotional support and helping them navigate the challenges of living with diabetes.
8. Documentation and Reporting: Maintaining accurate and detailed patient records, documenting education sessions, treatment plans, and progress made.
9. Professional Organizations: Active membership in professional organizations, such as the American Association of Diabetes Educators (AADE), can provide networking opportunities, access to resources, and continuing education opportunities.

Miscellaneous Information You Should Know

To enter the Diabetes Educator Nursing specialty, consider the following:

1. Gain Experience in Diabetes Care: Acquiring experience in diabetes management through clinical rotations, working in diabetes clinics, or seeking mentorship from experienced Diabetes Educator Nurses can provide valuable knowledge and skills.
2. Obtain Additional Education: Pursuing continuing education programs, workshops, or advanced degrees in diabetes management or

diabetes education can enhance your knowledge and expertise in this field.

3. Network and Collaborate: Building professional connections with diabetes specialists, educators, and healthcare professionals working in diabetes management can provide learning opportunities and potential job leads.

4. Volunteer or Join Support Groups: Volunteering or participating in diabetes support groups can help you gain insights into the challenges faced by individuals with diabetes and their families and enhance your ability to provide empathetic care.

5. Stay Updated: Keep up-to-date with the latest research, guidelines, and advancements in diabetes management through reputable sources, such as scientific journals, professional organizations, and conferences.

Entering the Diabetes Educator Nursing specialty allows you to make a significant impact on the lives of individuals with diabetes by empowering them with knowledge, skills, and support to effectively manage their condition.

| Lactation Consulting |

Lactation Consulting Nursing is a specialized field that focuses on providing breastfeeding support and education to new mothers and families. Lactation Consultants (LCs) are healthcare professionals who have in-depth knowledge and expertise in lactation, breastfeeding techniques, and infant feeding. They work closely with mothers to address breastfeeding challenges, provide guidance on proper latch and positioning, offer solutions to common breastfeeding issues, and promote the overall health and well-being of both mother and baby.

A Day in the Life

A typical day in the life of a Lactation Consultant may involve:

1. Patient Consultations: Meeting with expectant or new mothers to provide prenatal or postpartum breastfeeding education, assess breastfeeding difficulties, and develop individualized care plans.

2. Breastfeeding Support: Assisting mothers with proper latch and positioning techniques, observing breastfeeding sessions, and providing guidance on milk production, infant feeding cues, and establishing breastfeeding routines.

3. Education and Counseling: Providing information on breastfeeding benefits, breast milk storage and handling, weaning, and addressing common concerns such as low milk supply, nipple pain, or infant feeding difficulties.

4. Assessments and Evaluations: Conducting comprehensive assessments of mother and baby's overall health, including assessing infant weight gain, evaluating breastfeeding effectiveness, and identifying any underlying issues or medical conditions.

5. Problem Solving: Helping mothers troubleshoot and find solutions to breastfeeding challenges, such as resolving latch issues, managing engorgement, or addressing mastitis or other breastfeeding-related complications.

6. Collaborative Care: Working collaboratively with healthcare professionals, including pediatricians, obstetricians, midwives, and nurses, to provide coordinated care and ensure the best outcomes for mother and baby.

7. Documentation: Maintaining accurate and detailed records of patient consultations, assessments, care plans, and recommendations.

8. Follow-Up Support: Providing ongoing support and follow-up consultations to monitor progress, address concerns, and adjust care plans as needed.

9. Community Outreach and Education: Conducting breastfeeding

classes, support groups, or community workshops to promote breastfeeding awareness and educate the public on the benefits of breastfeeding.

10. Continuing Education: Engaging in continuous learning and professional development by attending conferences, workshops, and staying updated on current research and best practices in lactation consulting.

Degree(s) Required

To pursue a career in Lactation Consulting Nursing, a minimum of a Bachelor of Science in Nursing (BSN) degree is typically required. However, some positions or organizations may prefer or require a Master of Science in Nursing (MSN) degree with a focus on lactation or breastfeeding.

Salary

$66,640 - $110,930

Specialty Certifications Available or Needed

Specialty certification is highly recommended for Lactation Consultants. The International Board of Lactation Consultant Examiners (IBLCE) offers the International Board Certified Lactation Consultant (IBCLC) credential, which requires specific educational requirements, clinical experience, and successful completion of an examination. The IBCLC certification is widely recognized and considered the gold standard in the field.

Job Requirements

To work as a Lactation Consultant, consider the following job requirements:

1. Lactation Expertise: In-depth knowledge of lactation physiology, breastfeeding techniques, infant feeding cues, breast milk production, and common breastfeeding challenges.

2. Clinical Experience: Experience working in obstetric, neonatal, or pediatric settings, providing care to mothers and infants, and developing skills in assessing breastfeeding difficulties and providing appropriate interventions.

3. Communication and Counseling Skills: Excellent communication and counseling skills to effectively educate, support, and empathize with mothers and families, and provide guidance in a compassionate and non-judgmental manner.

4. Collaborative Approach: Ability to collaborate with a multidisciplinary team, including physicians, nurses, midwives, and lactation consultants, to ensure coordinated care for mothers and infants.

5. Empathy and Cultural Sensitivity: Understanding and respecting cultural, social, and individual differences when providing care, and adapting counseling and education to meet the unique needs of diverse populations.

6. Professionalism and Ethical Conduct: Adhering to professional and ethical standards, maintaining patient confidentiality, and promoting evidence-based practice in lactation consulting.

7. Continuing Education: Staying updated on current research, best practices, and advancements in lactation and breastfeeding through continuing education, attending conferences, and participating in relevant professional development activities.

Miscellaneous Information You Should Know

To enter the field of Lactation Consulting, consider the following:

1. Obtain Clinical Experience: Gaining experience in obstetric, neonatal, or pediatric settings that provide exposure to breastfeeding support and care can be beneficial.

2. Pursue Continuing Education: Completing courses or workshops specifically focused on lactation and breastfeeding, such as those approved by the International Board of Lactation Consultant Examiners (IBLCE), can help develop the necessary knowledge and skills.

3. Gain Practical Experience: Seek opportunities to gain practical experience in providing breastfeeding support through internships, volunteer work, or clinical rotations in settings that offer lactation services.

4. Networking: Connect with experienced Lactation Consultants, join professional organizations such as the International Lactation Consultant Association (ILCA) or local breastfeeding support groups, and seek mentorship opportunities to build relationships within the field.

5. Fulfill Certification Requirements: Meet the educational and clinical experience requirements set by the International Board of Lactation Consultant Examiners (IBLCE) to become eligible to sit for the IBCLC certification exam.

Lactation Consulting Nursing is a rewarding specialty that focuses on supporting and promoting successful breastfeeding and nurturing the bond between mother and baby. By providing education, counseling, and evidence-based interventions, Lactation Consultants play a crucial role in helping mothers achieve their breastfeeding goals and ensuring the health and well-being of both mother and child.

| Domestic Violence Nursing |

Domestic Violence Nursing, also known as Intimate Partner Violence (IPV) Nursing, is a specialized field that focuses on providing care and support to individuals who have experienced domestic violence. Domestic violence encompasses physical, sexual, emotional, and financial abuse within intimate relationships. Domestic Violence Nurses play a critical role in identifying, assessing, and assisting survivors of domestic violence, advocating for their safety and well-being, and collaborating with other healthcare professionals and community resources to address the complex needs of survivors.

A Day in the Life

A typical day in the life of a Domestic Violence Nurse may involve:

1. Assessment and Screening: Conducting comprehensive assessments and screenings to identify signs of domestic violence, including physical injuries, emotional trauma, and behavioral indicators.

2. Safety Planning: Collaborating with survivors to develop safety plans that address immediate safety concerns, including access to emergency shelters, legal protection orders, and community resources.

3. Forensic Documentation: Documenting injuries and collecting forensic evidence following protocols for legal purposes, if required.

4. Crisis Intervention: Providing immediate emotional support and crisis intervention to survivors, ensuring their physical and psychological well-being.

5. Medical Care and Treatment: Administering medical care, including wound care, STI testing, and treatment, pregnancy testing, and managing other health conditions resulting from domestic violence.

6. Referrals and Resource Coordination: Connecting survivors with community resources such as counseling services, legal aid, housing assistance, and support groups.

7. Advocacy: Advocating for survivors' rights and needs within the healthcare system and collaborating with interdisciplinary teams to ensure comprehensive care.

8. Documentation and Reporting: Maintaining accurate and detailed documentation of assessments, interventions, referrals, and any legal documentation in compliance with ethical and legal standards.

9. Education and Prevention: Conducting educational sessions for healthcare professionals, community organizations, and the public to raise awareness about domestic violence, its impact, and available resources.

10. Collaborative Partnerships: Collaborating with social workers, law enforcement agencies, legal professionals, and community organizations to

provide comprehensive care and support to survivors.

11. Ongoing Support: Providing long-term support to survivors by ensuring follow-up care, connecting them to ongoing counseling services, and monitoring their progress and safety.

Degree(s) Required

To pursue a career in Domestic Violence Nursing, a minimum of an Associate Degree in Nursing (ADN) or a Bachelor of Science in Nursing (BSN) is typically required. However, some employers may prefer or require a BSN due to the specialized nature of domestic violence nursing. Additionally, obtaining an advanced degree in nursing, such as a Master of Science in Nursing (MSN) or Doctor of Nursing Practice (DNP), can provide advanced knowledge and leadership opportunities in this field.

Salary

$66,640 - $110,930

Specialty Certifications Available or Needed

While there isn't a specific certification exclusively for Domestic Violence Nursing, there are certifications available that can enhance your knowledge and skills in addressing interpersonal violence and supporting survivors. Some relevant certifications include:

1. Sexual Assault Nurse Examiner (SANE): The SANE certification focuses on forensic nursing skills related to sexual assault, which can be applicable in cases of domestic violence that involve sexual violence.

2. Forensic Nurse-Certified (FN-C): The FN-C certification is offered by the International Association of Forensic Nurses (IAFN) and validates your expertise in forensic nursing, including collecting and preserving evidence in cases of interpersonal violence.

3. Certified Family Nurse Practitioner (FNP): Obtaining certification as an FNP can be beneficial for nurses providing comprehensive care to individuals and families affected by domestic violence, as it expands your scope of practice and allows for a more holistic approach to healthcare.

While not specific to Domestic Violence Nursing, these certifications can provide specialized knowledge and skills to support survivors of domestic violence effectively.

Job Requirements

To work as a Domestic Violence Nurse, consider the following job requirements:

1. Knowledge of Domestic Violence: Deep understanding of the dynamics of domestic violence, including risk factors, assessment strategies, safety planning, and available resources.

2. Empathy and Sensitivity: Ability to provide empathetic and non-judgmental care to survivors, demonstrating sensitivity to the trauma they have experienced.

3. Trauma-Informed Care: Knowledge and implementation of trauma-informed care principles when interacting with survivors, ensuring their physical and emotional safety throughout the healthcare process.

4. Interdisciplinary Collaboration: Collaboration with social workers, legal professionals, law enforcement agencies, and community organizations to ensure comprehensive care and support for survivors.

5. Cultural Competence: Awareness of cultural diversity and the intersectionality of identities when providing care to survivors from different backgrounds.

6. Confidentiality and Ethical Considerations: Adherence to ethical guidelines and legal regulations regarding confidentiality, mandatory reporting, and patient consent in cases of domestic violence.

7. Ongoing Education and Training: Engagement in continuing education to stay updated on best practices in domestic violence nursing, trauma-informed care, and legal considerations related to domestic violence.

8. Self-Care and Resilience: Practice self-care and develop resilience strategies to cope with the emotional demands of working with survivors of domestic violence.

Miscellaneous Information You Should Know

To enter the field of Domestic Violence Nursing, consider the following:

1. Gain Experience in Trauma or Emergency Care: Acquiring experience in settings that provide care for trauma or emergency patients, such as emergency departments, critical care units, or forensic nursing, can provide valuable skills and exposure to working with survivors of violence.

2. Attend Domestic Violence Training Programs: Participate in specialized training programs, workshops, or conferences related to domestic violence nursing, trauma-informed care, and legal aspects of domestic violence.

3. Volunteer or Intern: Seek opportunities to volunteer or intern with organizations that focus on domestic violence prevention and support services, such as domestic violence shelters, crisis hotlines, or advocacy groups.

4. Professional Organizations: Join professional organizations, such as the International Association of Forensic Nurses (IAFN) or local domestic

violence nursing associations, to network with other professionals in the field and access resources and educational opportunities.

Working as a Domestic Violence Nurse offers an opportunity to make a difference in the lives of survivors, advocating for their safety and well-being, and assisting them in their healing journey. It requires a compassionate and non-judgmental approach, as well as a commitment to ongoing education and awareness of the resources available to support survivors of domestic violence.

| Telehealth Nursing |

Telehealth Nursing is a specialty that focuses on providing healthcare services remotely through telecommunication technologies. It involves using digital platforms, video conferencing, telephone consultations, and other virtual tools to assess, diagnose, treat, educate, and support patients in their healthcare needs. Telehealth Nurses leverage technology to bridge the gap between healthcare providers and patients, delivering quality care and promoting patient well-being from a distance.

A Day in the Life

A day in the life of a Telehealth Nurse can vary depending on the specific telehealth setting and patient population they serve. Some common activities and responsibilities may include:

1. Patient Assessment: Conducting remote assessments of patients' health conditions, reviewing medical histories, and evaluating symptoms via video or phone consultations.

2. Care Coordination: Collaborating with healthcare teams to coordinate and manage patient care plans, including referrals, medication management, and follow-up appointments.

3. Remote Monitoring: Utilizing remote monitoring devices or technologies to track patients' vital signs, symptoms, or treatment progress and providing necessary guidance or interventions.

4. Health Education and Counseling: Providing patient education on various health topics, offering lifestyle recommendations, and answering questions regarding treatment plans, medications, or self-care practices.

5. Teletriage: Assessing patients' conditions and determining appropriate levels of care, guiding them to seek emergency care when necessary or providing non-urgent care advice remotely.

6. Documentation and Communication: Documenting patient interactions, treatment plans, and care interventions in electronic health records (EHRs), and effectively communicating with other healthcare providers or team members.

7. Technology Support: Familiarizing patients with telehealth platforms, troubleshooting technical issues, and ensuring a seamless telehealth experience for both patients and healthcare providers.

8. Ethical and Legal Considerations: Adhering to ethical guidelines, privacy regulations, and maintaining patient confidentiality during telehealth encounters.

9. Professional Development: Engaging in continuous learning and staying updated on telehealth best practices, new technologies, and emerging telehealth policies or regulations.

Degree(s) Required

To pursue a career in Telehealth Nursing, a minimum of a Bachelor of Science in Nursing (BSN) degree is typically required. However, some employers may consider registered nurses with an Associate Degree in Nursing (ADN) or diploma in nursing, combined with relevant experience and additional training in telehealth.

Salary

$65,210 - $106,830

Specialty Certifications Available or Needed

While there are no specific certifications exclusive to Telehealth Nursing, acquiring certifications in telehealth or related areas can enhance a nurse's knowledge and expertise in remote care delivery. Some relevant certifications include:

1. American Telemedicine Association (ATA) Certification: The ATA offers various certifications, including the Certified Telemedicine Clinical Presenter (CTCP) and the Certified Telehealth Coordinator (CTC), which validate proficiency in telehealth technologies, protocols, and best practices.

2. Telehealth Certification Institute (TCI) Certification: TCI provides certifications such as the Certified Clinical Telemental Health Provider (CCTMHP) and the Certified Clinical Telemental Health Supervisor (CCTMH-S), focusing on mental health services delivered via telehealth.

3. Vendor-Specific Certifications: Some telehealth technology vendors offer certifications specific to their platforms or equipment, providing specialized training in their use and application.

Job Requirements

To pursue a career in Telehealth Nursing, consider the following job requirements:

1. Nursing License: You must hold a valid registered nurse (RN) license in the state where you practice, ensuring compliance with nursing regulations and scope of practice guidelines.

2. Telehealth Knowledge and Skills: Familiarity with telehealth platforms, video conferencing tools, and electronic health record (EHR) systems, along with the ability to navigate and utilize these technologies effectively.

3. Clinical Experience: Prior experience in a clinical setting, such as medical-surgical, primary care, or specialty nursing, is valuable to provide a strong foundation in patient assessment, diagnosis, and treatment planning.

4. Communication Skills: Excellent verbal and written communication skills are essential to establish rapport with patients remotely, deliver clear instructions, and provide empathetic and compassionate care.

5. Critical Thinking and Decision-Making: Strong critical thinking abilities to assess patients remotely, identify urgent situations, and make appropriate clinical decisions within the telehealth context.

6. Adaptability and Flexibility: Telehealth environments can be dynamic and rapidly changing. Being adaptable and flexible to new technologies, workflows, and patient populations is crucial.

7. Regulatory and Legal Compliance: Knowledge of relevant telehealth regulations, privacy laws (e.g., HIPAA compliance), and state-specific guidelines governing remote care provision.

8. Cultural Competence: Sensitivity to diverse patient populations, cultural differences, and the ability to provide culturally competent care through remote interactions.

9. Professionalism and Ethics: Adhering to ethical principles, maintaining patient confidentiality, and practicing within the boundaries of the nursing profession and telehealth guidelines.

10. Continuous Learning: Keeping up-to-date with telehealth advancements, attending telehealth-specific training or conferences, and engaging in professional development opportunities.

Miscellaneous Information You Should Know

To enter the field of Telehealth Nursing, consider the following:

1. Telehealth Training: Seek additional training or courses in telehealth concepts, practices, and technologies to enhance your knowledge and proficiency in delivering remote care.

2. Networking and Collaboration: Connect with other Telehealth Nurses or professionals in the field to learn from their experiences, exchange best practices, and explore potential collaboration opportunities.

3. State-Specific Regulations: Familiarize yourself with telehealth regulations and licensing requirements specific to the state(s) where you intend to practice, as regulations may vary.

4. Telehealth Policies and Reimbursement: Stay updated with evolving telehealth policies, reimbursement models, and insurance coverage related to telehealth services.

5. Professional Associations: Join relevant professional associations or organizations focused on telehealth or telemedicine, such as the American Telemedicine Association (ATA), to access resources, networking opportunities, and industry updates.

6. Clinical Specialty Knowledge: Consider gaining expertise in a specific clinical area, such as mental health, primary care, or chronic disease

management, to provide specialized telehealth services.

7. Technology Proficiency: Stay current with telehealth technologies, including video conferencing platforms, remote monitoring devices, and mobile health applications, to effectively engage in remote patient care.

Becoming a Telehealth Nurse offers the opportunity to provide patient-centered care remotely, reach underserved populations, and contribute to expanding access to healthcare. It requires a blend of clinical nursing skills, technology proficiency, effective communication, and adaptability to deliver quality care through virtual means.

| Holistic Nursing |

Holistic Nursing is a specialty that focuses on providing care that integrates the physical, emotional, social, and spiritual aspects of individuals to promote their overall well-being. Holistic nurses consider the whole person and their unique needs, emphasizing the connection between mind, body, and spirit. They utilize complementary and alternative therapies along with conventional nursing approaches to support healing and promote holistic health.

A Day in the Life
A typical day in the life of a Holistic Nurse may involve:

1. Comprehensive Assessments: Conducting thorough assessments of patients' physical, emotional, social, and spiritual health to understand their holistic needs and develop individualized care plans.

2. Patient Education: Providing education and guidance to patients and their families on holistic health practices, self-care techniques, stress reduction, nutrition, exercise, and other wellness strategies.

3. Holistic Care Planning: Developing care plans that address the physical, emotional, social, and spiritual dimensions of patient well-being, integrating complementary therapies and conventional nursing interventions.

4. Complementary Therapies: Incorporating various holistic modalities into patient care, such as therapeutic touch, aromatherapy, meditation, guided imagery, acupuncture, herbal remedies, and energy healing.

5. Mind-Body-Spirit Connection: Recognizing and addressing the interconnectedness of physical, emotional, and spiritual health to promote healing and well-being.

6. Collaboration with Healthcare Team: Collaborating with other healthcare professionals, such as physicians, therapists, and counselors, to ensure a comprehensive approach to patient care.

7. Supportive Presence: Providing a compassionate and supportive presence for patients and their families, addressing their emotional and spiritual needs during times of illness, pain, or crisis.

8. Health Promotion: Promoting preventive care and empowering patients to take an active role in their health through healthy lifestyle choices and self-care practices.

9. Advocacy: Advocating for holistic approaches to healthcare and contributing to policy discussions and initiatives that support integrative and holistic nursing practices.

10. Personal Growth and Self-Care: Engaging in self-care practices, personal growth, and maintaining a holistic lifestyle to enhance one's own

well-being and serve as a role model for patients.

Degree(s) Required

To pursue a career in Holistic Nursing, a minimum of a Bachelor of Science in Nursing (BSN) degree is typically required. However, some positions or advanced roles may require a Master of Science in Nursing (MSN) or a graduate degree in Holistic Nursing or a related field. Advanced degrees provide a deeper understanding of holistic nursing concepts, research methodologies, and leadership skills.

Salary

$66,640 - $110,820

Specialty Certifications Available or Needed

While there is no specific certification for Holistic Nursing, nurses can pursue certifications in various complementary therapies or modalities to enhance their knowledge and practice. Some examples include:

1. Holistic Nursing Certification: The American Holistic Nurses Credentialing Corporation (AHNCC) offers certification as a Holistic Nurse (HN-BC) for nurses who meet specific education and practice requirements.
2. Certification in Therapeutic Modalities: Nurses can obtain certifications in specific complementary therapies such as aromatherapy, therapeutic touch, acupuncture, or herbal medicine through organizations or programs dedicated to those modalities.

These certifications demonstrate a nurse's commitment to holistic care and expertise in specific complementary therapies.

Job Requirements

To work as a Holistic Nurse, consider the following job requirements:

1. Holistic Nursing Knowledge: A solid understanding of holistic nursing principles, concepts, and modalities, including the mind-body-spirit connection and complementary therapies.
2. Holistic Assessment Skills: Proficiency in conducting comprehensive assessments that address physical, emotional, social, and spiritual aspects of patients' health.
3. Knowledge of Complementary Therapies: Familiarity with a range of complementary therapies and their application in nursing practice.
4. Patient-Centered Care: Ability to develop individualized care plans that align with patients' holistic needs, preferences, and values.

5. Collaboration and Communication: Strong communication and collaboration skills to work effectively with patients, families, and interdisciplinary healthcare teams.

6. Cultural Competence: Understanding and respecting diverse cultural beliefs, values, and practices related to health and healing.

7. Self-Care Practices: Engaging in personal self-care practices to maintain one's own well-being and serve as a role model for patients.

8. Continuous Learning: Commitment to staying updated with current research, evidence-based practices, and emerging trends in holistic nursing.

Miscellaneous Information You Should Know

To enter the field of Holistic Nursing, consider the following:

1. Holistic Approach Integration: Seek opportunities to incorporate holistic care principles into your current nursing practice and explore how complementary therapies can enhance patient outcomes.

2. Continuing Education: Attend workshops, conferences, and educational programs focused on holistic nursing, complementary therapies, and mind-body-spirit approaches.

3. Professional Organizations: Join professional organizations dedicated to holistic nursing, such as the American Holistic Nurses Association (AHNA), to connect with like-minded professionals, access resources, and stay updated with the latest developments in the field.

4. Networking and Mentorship: Connect with experienced holistic nurses who can provide guidance, support, and mentorship as you navigate your career in holistic nursing.

5. Personal Commitment: Cultivate your own holistic lifestyle and self-care practices, as they will not only benefit your own well-being but also enhance your ability to support patients on their healing journeys.

Holistic Nursing is a rewarding specialty that allows nurses to provide comprehensive and compassionate care, addressing the unique needs of individuals holistically. It requires a deep understanding of holistic principles, complementary therapies, and a commitment to ongoing learning and personal growth.

| Legal Nurse Consulting |

Legal Nurse Consulting is a specialized field where nurses apply their medical expertise and knowledge of healthcare to assist attorneys, insurance companies, and other legal professionals in navigating medical-related cases. Legal Nurse Consultants (LNCs) bridge the gap between healthcare and the legal system by analyzing medical records, providing expert opinions, and offering guidance on healthcare-related legal matters.

A Day in the Life

A typical day in the life of a Legal Nurse Consultant may involve:

1. Medical Record Review: Analyzing medical records, reports, and other relevant documents to identify medical issues, discrepancies, and potential areas of negligence or malpractice.

2. Case Research: Conducting extensive research on medical conditions, treatments, procedures, and relevant healthcare laws and regulations to support the legal team in building their case.

3. Expert Opinion Preparation: Providing expert opinions and insights based on nursing knowledge and experience to assist attorneys in understanding complex medical concepts and terminology.

4. Collaboration with Legal Team: Collaborating with attorneys, paralegals, and other legal professionals to develop case strategies, identify key witnesses, and prepare for depositions or trials.

5. Medical Expert Witness Support: Assisting in the selection and preparation of medical expert witnesses for testimony, including reviewing their qualifications and helping with the formulation of questions.

6. Medical Literature Review: Staying up-to-date with current medical research, advancements, and evidence-based practices relevant to ongoing cases.

7. Consultation and Communication: Participating in meetings, conferences, and consultations with clients, attorneys, and medical professionals to discuss case details, medical issues, and legal strategies.

8. Report Writing: Compiling detailed reports summarizing medical findings, assessments, and interpretations in a clear and concise manner that can be easily understood by legal professionals.

9. Deposition and Trial Support: Providing support during depositions and trials, including assisting in the preparation of witnesses, analyzing testimony, and helping to present medical evidence effectively.

10. Continuing Education: Engaging in ongoing professional development, attending legal nurse consulting seminars, workshops, and conferences to enhance knowledge and skills in both the healthcare and legal domains.

Degree(s) Required

To pursue a career in Legal Nurse Consulting, a minimum of a Bachelor of Science in Nursing (BSN) degree is typically required. However, some positions or advanced roles may prefer or require a Master of Science in Nursing (MSN) degree or a legal nurse consulting certificate program.

Salary

$67,010 - $121,630

Specialty Certifications Available or Needed

While not mandatory, obtaining certification as a Legal Nurse Consultant can enhance professional credibility and demonstrate specialized knowledge. The American Association of Legal Nurse Consultants (AALNC) offers the Legal Nurse Consultant Certified (LNCC) credential, which requires meeting specific educational and experience requirements and passing an examination.

Job Requirements

To work as a Legal Nurse Consultant, consider the following job requirements:

1. Nursing Expertise: Extensive clinical experience and expertise in a nursing specialty, allowing for a comprehensive understanding of medical practices, procedures, terminology, and healthcare delivery systems.

2. Knowledge of Legal and Regulatory Framework: Understanding of relevant laws, regulations, and legal processes related to healthcare, medical malpractice, personal injury, product liability, or other areas of legal focus.

3. Analytical and Critical Thinking Skills: Strong analytical and critical thinking abilities to evaluate medical records, identify relevant medical issues, and provide accurate assessments and opinions.

4. Communication and Interpersonal Skills: Effective communication skills, both written and verbal, to convey complex medical concepts and opinions clearly and professionally to legal professionals and non-medical audiences.

5. Attention to Detail: Meticulous attention to detail when reviewing medical records and conducting research, ensuring accuracy and completeness of information.

6. Legal Research Skills: Proficiency in conducting legal research, identifying relevant case laws, statutes, regulations, and other legal resources related to specific cases.

7. Ethical and Professional Conduct: Adhering to professional and ethical standards, maintaining confidentiality, and avoiding conflicts of

interest.

8. Continuing Education: Keeping up-to-date with changes in healthcare practices, regulations, and legal requirements through continuous learning and professional development.

Miscellaneous Information You Should Know

To enter the field of Legal Nurse Consulting, consider the following:

1. Gaining Clinical Experience: Building a strong foundation of clinical nursing experience in a specific specialty is beneficial as it provides a deeper understanding of medical practices and procedures.

2. Networking: Connecting with legal professionals, attending legal conferences, joining legal nurse consulting associations, and establishing professional relationships can help create opportunities in the field.

3. Legal Knowledge: Developing a basic understanding of legal principles, terminology, and processes through self-study or legal-related courses can be advantageous.

4. Legal Nurse Consulting Courses: Completing legal nurse consulting courses or certification programs can enhance knowledge and skills specific to this field and increase employability.

5. Professional Associations: Joining professional associations such as the American Association of Legal Nurse Consultants (AALNC) can provide networking opportunities, access to resources, and educational support.

Legal Nurse Consulting is a unique nursing specialty that allows nurses to apply their healthcare expertise in a legal context. It requires a strong understanding of both nursing and the legal system, analytical skills, and effective communication to support attorneys and legal professionals in healthcare-related cases.

| Genetics Counseling Nursing |

Genetics Counseling Nursing, also known as Genetic Nursing or Genetic Counseling, is a specialized field that combines genetics, counseling, and nursing to provide comprehensive care to individuals and families with genetic conditions or at risk of inherited disorders. Genetics counselors work closely with patients to assess their risk, provide information about genetic conditions, facilitate genetic testing, and offer emotional support and guidance in making informed decisions about their healthcare. They play a crucial role in promoting genetic literacy, empowering individuals and families to understand and navigate the complexities of genetic information.

A Day in the Life

A typical day in the life of a Genetics Counseling Nurse may involve:

1. Patient Assessment: Conducting comprehensive assessments of patients' medical history, family history, and genetic risk factors to identify potential genetic conditions or inherited disorders.

2. Genetic Counseling: Providing genetic counseling sessions to patients and families, discussing the nature of genetic conditions, assessing their impact on individuals and families, and addressing their emotional, psychological, and ethical concerns.

3. Risk Assessment and Education: Evaluating the likelihood of genetic conditions or inherited disorders based on family history, genetic testing results, and other relevant factors. Educating patients about their genetic risk, inheritance patterns, and available preventive or treatment options.

4. Genetic Testing Coordination: Facilitating genetic testing, including ordering appropriate tests, explaining the process and implications, and helping patients understand and interpret the results.

5. Interdisciplinary Collaboration: Collaborating with geneticists, physicians, nurses, and other healthcare professionals to develop individualized care plans and coordinate ongoing care for patients with genetic conditions.

6. Patient Advocacy: Advocating for patients' needs, rights, and access to appropriate genetic services, resources, and support groups.

7. Research and Education: Staying updated on advances in genetics and genetic counseling through research, continuing education, and professional development activities. Participating in educational initiatives to increase genetic literacy among healthcare professionals and the general public.

8. Ethical and Legal Considerations: Ensuring compliance with ethical guidelines, informed consent processes, and legal regulations related to genetic counseling and patient privacy.

Degree(s) Required

To pursue a career in Genetics Counseling Nursing, a Master's degree in Genetic Counseling or a related field is typically required. Programs accredited by the Accreditation Council for Genetic Counseling (ACGC) are recommended, as they provide the necessary education and clinical training to become a licensed genetics counselor. The Master's program typically takes two to three years to complete and includes coursework in genetics, counseling theory, psychosocial aspects of genetics, and clinical rotations in genetics clinics.

Salary

$70,670 - $120,690

Specialty Certifications Available or Needed

After completing the required education, genetics counselors can obtain certification through the American Board of Genetic Counseling (ABGC). Certification as a Certified Genetic Counselor (CGC) demonstrates competency in the field and is often required or preferred by employers. To maintain certification, ongoing continuing education is necessary.

Job Requirements

To work as a Genetics Counseling Nurse, consider the following job requirements:

1. Strong Knowledge of Genetics: A solid understanding of genetics principles, genetic conditions, inheritance patterns, and genetic testing methodologies.
2. Counseling and Communication Skills: Excellent communication and counseling skills to effectively communicate complex genetic information, provide emotional support, and empower patients and families to make informed decisions.
3. Empathy and Sensitivity: Ability to empathize with individuals and families facing genetic challenges, showing sensitivity to their emotions, cultural background, and personal beliefs.
4. Ethical and Professional Conduct: Adherence to ethical guidelines and legal regulations governing genetic counseling, patient privacy, and informed consent.
5. Interdisciplinary Collaboration: The ability to collaborate with a multidisciplinary team of healthcare professionals, including geneticists, physicians, nurses, and psychologists, to ensure comprehensive patient care.
6. Continuing Education: A commitment to ongoing learning and professional development to stay updated on advancements in genetics and genetic counseling.

7. Emotional Resilience: The capacity to handle emotionally challenging situations and provide support to individuals and families coping with genetic conditions or difficult decisions.

Miscellaneous Information You Should Know

To enter the field of Genetics Counseling Nursing, consider the following:

1. Gain Clinical Experience: Many genetic counseling programs require applicants to have relevant clinical experience, such as in genetics clinics, research labs, or healthcare settings.

2. Research Genetic Counseling Programs: Look for accredited genetic counseling programs that provide comprehensive training and clinical rotations in genetics clinics.

3. Volunteer or Shadowing Opportunities: Seek opportunities to volunteer or shadow genetic counselors to gain firsthand experience and insight into the field.

4. Professional Organizations: Join professional organizations such as the National Society of Genetic Counselors (NSGC) to access resources, networking opportunities, and mentorship programs.

5. Certification Exam Preparation: Prepare for the certification exam administered by the American Board of Genetic Counseling by reviewing study materials and participating in practice exams.

Working as a Genetics Counseling Nurse allows you to combine your expertise in genetics and nursing with counseling skills to provide essential support to individuals and families facing genetic conditions. It requires a strong knowledge of genetics, effective communication and counseling abilities, and the ability to navigate complex ethical and legal considerations.

| Nurse Entrepreneur |

Nurse Entrepreneurs are registered nurses who have taken on entrepreneurial ventures, utilizing their nursing background and expertise to start and operate their own businesses or ventures within the healthcare industry. Nurse Entrepreneurs combine their clinical knowledge, healthcare skills, and business acumen to identify gaps in healthcare services, develop innovative solutions, and provide unique products or services to meet the needs of patients, healthcare organizations, or other target markets.

A Day in the Life

A day in the life of a Nurse Entrepreneur can vary greatly depending on the specific business or venture they have established. Some common activities and responsibilities may include:

1. Business Planning: Developing and refining business plans, including market analysis, financial projections, and operational strategies.

2. Product or Service Development: Creating and refining unique products, services, or programs that align with the target market's needs and address healthcare challenges or gaps.

3. Marketing and Promotion: Implementing marketing strategies, including branding, advertising, and online presence, to reach and attract clients or customers.

4. Client or Customer Engagement: Building and maintaining relationships with clients or customers, understanding their needs, and providing exceptional customer service.

5. Operations Management: Overseeing day-to-day operations, managing finances, coordinating logistics, and ensuring regulatory compliance.

6. Networking and Collaboration: Establishing professional networks, collaborating with other healthcare professionals or organizations, and seeking partnerships or collaborations to enhance business opportunities.

7. Continuous Learning: Staying updated with the latest trends, research, and innovations in the healthcare industry and incorporating relevant knowledge into business practices.

8. Business Growth and Development: Identifying opportunities for expansion, diversification, or scaling the business, including exploring new markets or introducing new products or services.

9. Financial Management: Monitoring financial performance, managing budgets, and seeking funding or investment opportunities to support business growth.

10. Leadership and Decision Making: Making strategic decisions, leading a team if applicable, and managing the overall direction and vision of the

business.

Degree(s) Required

The degree requirements for Nurse Entrepreneurs may vary depending on the nature of their business or venture. Generally, a minimum of a Bachelor of Science in Nursing (BSN) degree is recommended to establish a solid foundation in nursing practice, healthcare principles, and patient care. However, additional degrees such as a Master of Science in Nursing (MSN), Master of Business Administration (MBA), or other related fields can provide a broader skill set and business acumen to succeed as a Nurse Entrepreneur.

Salary

$65,300 - $126,740

Specialty Certifications Available or Needed

While there are no specific certifications exclusive to Nurse Entrepreneurs, acquiring certifications in specialized areas related to the business venture can add credibility and enhance the entrepreneur's expertise. For example, if the Nurse Entrepreneur operates a business focused on a specific healthcare specialty, such as wound care or diabetes management, certifications in those areas may be beneficial.

Job Requirements

To pursue a career as a Nurse Entrepreneur, consider the following job requirements:

1. Nursing Experience: Prior clinical experience as a registered nurse is valuable in establishing credibility, understanding healthcare challenges, and identifying potential business opportunities.

2. Business and Entrepreneurial Skills: A strong understanding of business principles, including marketing, finance, operations, and management, to effectively launch and manage a business.

3. Innovation and Creativity: The ability to think outside the box, identify unmet needs, and develop innovative solutions or products that can improve healthcare delivery or address healthcare gaps.

4. Communication and Networking: Excellent communication skills to effectively promote products or services, build professional networks, and establish collaborations with relevant stakeholders.

5. Financial Management: Basic knowledge of financial management, budgeting, and revenue generation to ensure the financial sustainability of the business.

6. Problem-Solving and Decision-Making: Strong problem-solving skills

to overcome challenges, make critical business decisions, and adapt to the evolving healthcare landscape.

7. Entrepreneurial Mindset: Possessing an entrepreneurial spirit, including traits such as risk-taking, resilience, self-motivation, and a willingness to embrace uncertainty.

8. Regulatory and Legal Compliance: Understanding and adhering to relevant healthcare regulations, licensing requirements, and legal obligations associated with the business venture.

9. Continuous Learning: Commitment to ongoing professional development, staying updated with industry trends, healthcare advancements, and business strategies through courses, workshops, or self-directed learning.

Miscellaneous Information You Should Know

Entering the field of Nurse Entrepreneurship involves a combination of nursing knowledge and business acumen. Consider the following:

1. Identify a Niche: Determine your specific area of interest or expertise within the healthcare industry and identify potential gaps or opportunities that can be addressed through entrepreneurial endeavors.

2. Business Plan Development: Develop a comprehensive business plan that outlines the mission, vision, target market, competition analysis, marketing strategies, financial projections, and operational framework.

3. Networking and Mentorship: Build a network of other Nurse Entrepreneurs, healthcare professionals, or business experts who can provide guidance, support, and mentorship throughout your entrepreneurial journey.

4. Seek Professional Development: Consider pursuing additional education, training, or certifications in business management, entrepreneurship, marketing, or any other relevant areas to strengthen your business skills and knowledge.

5. Start Small and Scale Up: Begin with a well-defined and manageable business concept, validate its feasibility, and gradually expand and diversify as you gain experience and establish a solid foundation.

6. Embrace Technology: Stay updated with technological advancements in the healthcare industry and leverage digital tools, online platforms, and social media to enhance your business reach and efficiency.

7. Risk Management: Assess potential risks and develop strategies to mitigate them, such as obtaining appropriate insurance coverage and seeking legal counsel when necessary.

8. Collaborate and Partner: Explore opportunities to collaborate with healthcare organizations, community agencies, or other stakeholders to enhance your business offerings and reach a wider audience.

9. Continuously Evaluate and Adapt: Regularly assess the market, customer feedback, and business performance to make informed decisions, adapt to changing healthcare trends, and optimize your business model.

Becoming a Nurse Entrepreneur offers the opportunity to combine nursing expertise with business innovation, allowing for creativity, autonomy, and the potential to make a significant impact on healthcare delivery and patient outcomes. It requires a strong entrepreneurial mindset, a passion for improving healthcare, and a willingness to take calculated risks in pursuit of professional and personal fulfillment.

PART III:

PUBLIC HEALTH/COMMUNITY/GOVERNMENT SPECIALTIES

| Public Health Nursing |

Public health nursing is a specialized field that focuses on promoting and protecting the health of populations and communities. Public health nurses work to prevent disease, improve health outcomes, and address health disparities by implementing health promotion strategies, conducting community assessments, and providing direct care and education to individuals and groups. They work in a variety of settings, including government health agencies, community health centers, schools, and non-profit organizations.

A Day in the Life

A typical day in the life of a public health nurse may involve:

1. Assessing Public Health: Conducting community assessments to identify health needs, concerns, and existing resources. Collecting and analyzing data on health indicators, disease prevalence, and social determinants of health.

2. Health Promotion and Education: Developing and implementing health promotion programs and initiatives, such as immunization campaigns, prenatal education, chronic disease management, or substance abuse prevention. Delivering educational sessions and workshops to individuals and community groups.

3. Disease Prevention and Control: Collaborating with epidemiologists and other public health professionals to investigate disease outbreaks, track communicable diseases, and implement control measures. Providing guidance on infection prevention, contact tracing, and immunization protocols.

4. Policy Development: Participating in the development and evaluation of public health policies and guidelines at the local, state, or national level. Advocating for evidence-based practices and policies that improve population health.

5. Collaboration and Partnerships: Collaborating with community organizations, healthcare providers, and stakeholders to develop partnerships and promote health initiatives. Building coalitions to address community health needs and disparities.

6. Direct Patient Care: Providing direct care to individuals and families in homes, schools, or community health centers. Conducting health screenings, administering vaccinations, managing chronic conditions, and providing counseling and referrals.

7. Emergency Preparedness: Participating in emergency preparedness and response activities, including disaster planning, coordinating community resources during emergencies, and providing

healthcare services in crisis situations.

8. Data Collection and Evaluation: Collecting, analyzing, and interpreting health data to identify trends, assess program effectiveness, and make data-driven decisions. Monitoring and evaluating the impact of public health interventions.

9. Health Equity and Advocacy: Addressing health disparities and advocating for equitable access to healthcare services. Working to reduce barriers to care and improve health outcomes for marginalized populations.

10. Education and Professional Development: Engaging in continuous education to stay updated on current public health issues, evidence-based practices, and policies. Participating in conferences, workshops, and trainings to enhance knowledge and skills in public health nursing.

Degree(s) Required

To become a public health nurse, you need to earn a degree in nursing. The two common degree paths are an Associate Degree in Nursing (ADN) or a Bachelor of Science in Nursing (BSN). However, a BSN is increasingly preferred for public health nursing positions due to the comprehensive knowledge and leadership skills gained. Some public health nursing roles may require a Master of Public Health (MPH) degree or a related advanced nursing degree for leadership or research positions.

Salary
$61,700 - $91,820

Specialty Certifications Available or Needed

Certification in public health nursing can demonstrate specialized knowledge and competence. The American Nurses Credentialing Center (ANCC) offers the Public Health Nursing-Advanced (PHNA-BC) credential. Eligibility for the PHNA-BC certification typically requires a combination of education, clinical experience in public health nursing, and successful completion of an exam.

Job Requirements

Public health nursing requires a strong foundation in nursing practice, as well as additional knowledge and skills specific to population health. Job requirements may include:

1. Knowledge of public health principles, epidemiology, health promotion strategies, and evidence-based practices.
2. Understanding of community health assessment methods, including data collection, analysis, and interpretation.

3. Proficiency in health education and counseling techniques to provide effective health promotion and disease prevention interventions.

4. Familiarity with health policy and the ability to advocate for public health initiatives at various levels.

5. Collaboration with interdisciplinary teams and community stakeholders to develop and implement community health programs and policies.

6. Ability to work with diverse populations and address health disparities by applying cultural sensitivity and understanding.

7. Strong communication and interpersonal skills to effectively engage and educate individuals and communities about health issues.

8. Data management and evaluation skills to monitor health outcomes, assess program effectiveness, and make data-informed decisions.

9. Knowledge of emergency preparedness and response protocols to address public health emergencies and disasters.

10. Ability to stay updated with current research, evidence-based practices, and public health regulations and guidelines.

Miscellaneous Information You Should Know

To enter the public health nursing specialty, you may consider the following:

1. Gain experience in community or public health settings: Seek opportunities to gain experience in community health clinics, public health departments, or non-profit organizations focused on public health initiatives. This experience will provide valuable exposure to population health principles and community-based interventions.

2. Pursue additional education or certifications in public health: Consider pursuing a Master of Public Health (MPH) degree or a related advanced nursing degree with a public health focus. These programs provide in-depth knowledge of public health concepts, research methodologies, and leadership skills.

3. Volunteer or participate in community health projects: Engage in volunteer work or community health projects to gain practical experience in public health nursing. This involvement demonstrates your commitment to the field and allows you to apply public health principles in real-world settings.

4. Stay updated with public health issues and policies: Stay informed about current public health issues, research, and policies by accessing resources provided by professional organizations, such as the American Public Health Association (APHA) and the Centers for Disease Control and Prevention (CDC).

5. Networking and professional involvement: Engage with professional

organizations and networks focused on public health nursing to connect with other public health nurses, access educational resources, and stay informed about career opportunities. Participate in conferences, webinars, or local chapter meetings to expand your knowledge and network with professionals in the field.

Remember that specific requirements and preferences may vary depending on the healthcare organization, geographical location, and level of experience desired for public health nursing positions.

| Community Health Nursing |

Community health nursing focuses on promoting and maintaining the health of individuals, families, and communities through education, prevention, and coordination of healthcare services. Community health nurses work in diverse settings, such as public health departments, clinics, schools, and community organizations. They assess community health needs, develop and implement health promotion programs, provide direct care, and collaborate with community stakeholders to improve health outcomes.

A Day in the Life

A typical day in the life of a community health nurse may involve:

1. Assessing Community Health: Conducting community assessments to identify health needs, concerns, and existing resources. Collecting and analyzing data on health indicators, disease prevalence, and social determinants of health.

2. Health Promotion and Education: Developing and implementing health promotion programs and initiatives, such as immunization campaigns, prenatal education, chronic disease management, or substance abuse prevention. Delivering educational sessions and workshops to individuals and community groups.

3. Disease Prevention and Control: Collaborating with epidemiologists and other public health professionals to investigate disease outbreaks, track communicable diseases, and implement control measures. Providing guidance on infection prevention, contact tracing, and immunization protocols.

4. Policy Development: Participating in the development and evaluation of public health policies and guidelines at the local, state, or national level. Advocating for evidence-based practices and policies that improve population health.

5. Collaboration and Partnerships: Collaborating with community organizations, healthcare providers, and stakeholders to develop partnerships and promote health initiatives. Building coalitions to address community health needs and disparities.

6. Direct Patient Care: Providing direct care to individuals and families in homes, schools, or community health centers. Conducting health screenings, administering vaccinations, managing chronic conditions, and providing counseling and referrals.

7. Emergency Preparedness: Participating in emergency preparedness and response activities, including disaster planning, coordinating community resources during emergencies, and providing

healthcare services in crisis situations.

8. Data Collection and Evaluation: Collecting, analyzing, and interpreting health data to identify trends, assess program effectiveness, and make data-driven decisions. Monitoring and evaluating the impact of public health interventions.

9. Health Equity and Advocacy: Addressing health disparities and advocating for equitable access to healthcare services. Working to reduce barriers to care and improve health outcomes for marginalized populations.

10. Education and Professional Development: Engaging in continuous education to stay updated on current public health issues, evidence-based practices, and policies. Participating in conferences, workshops, and trainings to enhance knowledge and skills in public health nursing.

Degree(s) Required

To become a community health nurse, you need to earn a degree in nursing. The two common degree paths are an Associate Degree in Nursing (ADN) or a Bachelor of Science in Nursing (BSN). However, pursuing a Bachelor's degree is increasingly preferred in community health nursing due to the comprehensive knowledge and leadership skills gained. Additionally, pursuing a Master of Public Health (MPH) or a Master of Science in Nursing (MSN) with a specialization in community health nursing can provide advanced training and career opportunities in this field.

Salary
$61,700 - $91,810

Specialty Certifications Available or Needed

Certification in community health nursing can demonstrate specialized knowledge and commitment to the specialty. The American Nurses Credentialing Center (ANCC) offers the Advanced Public Health Nursing-Board Certified (APHN-BC) credential, which validates expertise in community health nursing. Eligibility for the APHN-BC certification typically requires a combination of education and experience in community health nursing.

Job Requirements

Community health nursing requires strong assessment, communication, and advocacy skills, as well as the ability to work independently and within a multidisciplinary team. Job requirements may include:

1. Proficiency in community health assessment, including analyzing

epidemiological data and identifying health needs and priorities.

2. Skill in developing and implementing health promotion and disease prevention programs for individuals and communities.

3. Knowledge of community resources, healthcare systems, and public health policies.

4. Ability to provide direct care and health education to individuals and families in diverse community settings.

5. Competence in collaborating with community stakeholders, such as government agencies, nonprofits, schools, and community organizations.

6. Effective communication and cultural competence to engage with diverse populations and address health disparities.

Miscellaneous Information You Should Know

To enter the community health nursing specialty, you may consider the following:

1. Gain experience in community settings: Acquiring experience in community health settings, such as public health departments, community clinics, or nonprofit organizations, can provide valuable insights into the unique challenges and opportunities in community health nursing. Seek internships, volunteer opportunities, or employment in community health-related roles.

2. Pursue additional education or certifications: Consider pursuing additional education or certifications specific to community health nursing. This may include a Master's degree in Public Health (MPH) or a certificate program in community health. These programs can provide specialized knowledge in population health, health promotion, and community assessment.

3. Stay updated with public health practices and policies: Community health nursing is influenced by evolving public health practices and policies. Stay informed about public health guidelines, epidemiological trends, and health promotion strategies through professional organizations, journals, and continuing education programs focused on community health.

4. Develop strong communication and cultural competence: Effective communication and cultural competence are essential in community health nursing. Enhance your communication skills to engage with diverse populations, build rapport, and facilitate health education. Cultural competence helps address health disparities and promote equitable healthcare.

5. Networking and collaboration: Engage with professional organizations like the Public Health Nursing Section of the American Public Health Association (APHA) to connect with community health professionals, access resources, and stay informed about emerging practices.

Collaborate with community stakeholders, such as local health departments or community-based organizations, to establish relationships and gain practical experience.

Remember that specific requirements and preferences may vary depending on the healthcare organization, geographical location, and level of experience desired for community health nursing positions.

| Global Health Nursing |

Global Health Nursing is a specialized field that focuses on addressing health disparities, promoting health equity, and improving healthcare outcomes on a global scale. Nurses working in global health play a crucial role in delivering healthcare services, implementing health programs, and advocating for policies that address the unique healthcare needs of underserved populations and communities around the world. They may work in international organizations, non-governmental organizations (NGOs), government agencies, or academic institutions, collaborating with local healthcare providers and communities to improve access to quality healthcare, prevent diseases, and enhance overall health outcomes.

A Day in the Life

A typical day in the life of a Global Health Nurse may involve:

1. Community Assessments: Conducting assessments of communities' health needs, identifying prevalent health issues, and determining priorities for intervention.

2. Health Promotion and Education: Developing and implementing health promotion programs, providing education on disease prevention, hygiene practices, reproductive health, nutrition, and other relevant topics to individuals and communities.

3. Capacity Building: Collaborating with local healthcare providers and community members to enhance their knowledge and skills in healthcare delivery, public health, and health system strengthening.

4. Program Planning and Management: Designing and managing global health programs, including developing goals and objectives, coordinating activities, monitoring progress, and evaluating outcomes.

5. Clinical Care and Health Services: Providing direct patient care, often in resource-limited settings, by addressing acute and chronic health conditions, performing screenings, administering vaccinations, and managing primary healthcare needs.

6. Cultural Sensitivity and Adaptation: Respecting and understanding the cultural, social, and economic factors influencing healthcare practices and tailoring interventions to local contexts.

7. Collaboration and Partnerships: Working closely with local healthcare providers, government agencies, NGOs, and other stakeholders to foster collaboration, strengthen healthcare systems, and advocate for policy changes that improve health outcomes.

8. Research and Data Analysis: Conducting research projects, collecting and analyzing data, and contributing to evidence-based practices and policies in global health.

9. Emergency Response and Disaster Relief: Participating in emergency response efforts, providing healthcare services and support during natural disasters, epidemics, or humanitarian crises.

10. Advocacy and Policy Development: Advocating for improved health policies, equitable access to healthcare resources, and social determinants of health at local, national, and international levels.

Degree(s) Required

To pursue a career in Global Health Nursing, a Bachelor of Science in Nursing (BSN) is typically required. However, higher-level degrees such as Master of Science in Nursing (MSN) or Doctor of Nursing Practice (DNP) with a focus on global health or public health can provide advanced knowledge and skills in this field. Additional training and education in global health, public health, or international development can also be beneficial.

Salary

$61,700 - $91,800

Specialty Certifications Available or Needed

While there isn't a specific certification for Global Health Nursing, obtaining certifications in related areas such as Public Health Nursing or International Health may enhance your knowledge and skills. Certification options include Certified in Public Health (CPH) or Certified Public Health Nurse (CPHN), which demonstrate expertise in public health principles and practices.

Job Requirements

To work in Global Health Nursing, consider the following job requirements:

1. Knowledge of Global Health Issues: Understanding global health challenges, social determinants of health, cultural competency, and health disparities across different populations and regions.

2. Strong Communication Skills: Effective communication and cross-cultural communication skills to work with diverse populations, collaborate with local healthcare providers, and advocate for health equity.

3. Flexibility and Adaptability: Ability to adapt to different healthcare systems, resource-limited environments, and cultural contexts.

4. Research and Data Analysis: Proficiency in research methodologies, data collection, analysis, and interpretation to inform evidence-based practices and policies.

5. Program Management: Skills in planning, implementing, and

managing global health programs, including budgeting, monitoring, and evaluation.

6. Collaboration and Partnerships: The ability to work collaboratively with local communities, government agencies, NGOs, and other stakeholders to achieve common goals.

7. Leadership and Advocacy: Capacity to lead global health initiatives, advocate for policy changes, and drive health system improvements.

8. Willingness to Travel: Global Health Nurses often work in diverse settings and may be required to travel frequently or live in different countries for extended periods.

9. Multilingual Skills: Proficiency in additional languages relevant to the populations or regions of focus can be advantageous.

Miscellaneous Information You Should Know

To enter the field of Global Health Nursing, consider the following:

1. Gain Clinical Experience: Obtain clinical experience in diverse healthcare settings, preferably with exposure to international or cross-cultural populations.

2. Pursue Additional Education: Consider pursuing a Master's degree or specialized training in global health, public health, or international development to enhance your expertise in the field.

3. Seek Field Experience: Look for opportunities to engage in international or global health projects, fieldwork, or volunteer programs that provide direct exposure to global health challenges and best practices.

4. Join Professional Organizations: Join global health organizations, such as the Consortium of Universities for Global Health (CUGH) or Global Health Council, to access networking opportunities, resources, and career development support.

5. Stay Updated: Keep up with current research, emerging trends, and global health policies through publications, conferences, and online platforms focused on global health.

Working in Global Health Nursing allows you to make a significant impact on healthcare disparities, improve health outcomes, and contribute to global health initiatives. It requires a strong understanding of global health issues, effective communication and collaboration skills, and the ability to adapt to diverse healthcare settings and cultural contexts.

| Lifestyle and Wellness Nursing |

Lifestyle and Wellness Nursing is a specialized field that focuses on promoting health and well-being through lifestyle interventions, health education, and disease prevention strategies. Lifestyle and Wellness Nurses work with individuals, families, and communities to assess their health needs, develop personalized wellness plans, and empower them to make positive lifestyle choices. They provide guidance on nutrition, physical activity, stress management, smoking cessation, and other lifestyle factors that impact overall health.

A Day in the Life

A typical day in the life of a Lifestyle and Wellness Nurse may involve:

1. Health Assessments: Conducting comprehensive health assessments, including lifestyle and wellness evaluations, to identify risk factors and develop personalized wellness plans.

2. Health Education: Providing individual or group health education sessions on topics such as nutrition, exercise, stress management, sleep hygiene, and smoking cessation.

3. Lifestyle Interventions: Collaborating with individuals and families to set realistic health goals and develop action plans for making sustainable lifestyle changes.

4. Counseling and Coaching: Offering counseling and coaching services to support behavior change, address barriers, and provide ongoing motivation and support.

5. Community Outreach: Engaging in community health promotion activities, organizing wellness workshops, and participating in health fairs to educate the public on healthy lifestyle choices.

6. Collaboration with Healthcare Providers: Working collaboratively with other healthcare professionals, such as physicians, dietitians, psychologists, and physical therapists, to provide holistic care and ensure coordinated support for individuals and communities.

7. Evaluation and Monitoring: Assessing the progress of individuals in achieving their health goals, monitoring their adherence to lifestyle changes, and making necessary adjustments to the wellness plans.

8. Documentation: Maintaining accurate and detailed records of assessments, education sessions, interventions, and progress reports.

9. Program Development: Participating in the development and implementation of wellness programs and initiatives within healthcare settings, schools, workplaces, or community organizations.

10. Professional Development: Staying updated on the latest

research, best practices, and evidence-based interventions in lifestyle and wellness nursing through continuing education, workshops, and professional conferences.

Degree(s) Required

To pursue a career in Lifestyle and Wellness Nursing, a minimum of a Bachelor of Science in Nursing (BSN) degree is typically required. However, some positions or organizations may prefer or require a Master of Science in Nursing (MSN) degree with a focus on lifestyle and wellness promotion.

Salary

$66,640 - $110,930

Specialty Certifications Available or Needed

While there are no specific certifications exclusively for Lifestyle and Wellness Nursing, obtaining certifications in related areas can enhance expertise in lifestyle interventions and health promotion. Examples include certifications in health coaching, nutrition counseling, smoking cessation counseling, or stress management coaching. Additionally, obtaining certification as a Wellness Coach from an accredited organization can provide additional credibility and demonstrate specialized knowledge in the field.

Job Requirements

To work as a Lifestyle and Wellness Nurse, consider the following job requirements:

1. Knowledge of Lifestyle Factors: In-depth understanding of lifestyle factors that impact health and wellness, such as nutrition, physical activity, stress management, sleep, and substance abuse.

2. Health Education and Counseling Skills: Effective communication and counseling skills to educate individuals and communities about lifestyle choices, provide guidance on behavior change, and motivate individuals to adopt healthy habits.

3. Health Assessment and Evaluation: Competence in conducting comprehensive health assessments, including lifestyle assessments, and evaluating individuals' progress in achieving health goals.

4. Knowledge of Evidence-Based Interventions: Familiarity with evidence-based interventions and strategies for promoting healthy lifestyles and preventing chronic diseases.

5. Cultural Competence: Awareness and respect for cultural, social, and individual differences when providing education and support, and the

ability to tailor interventions to meet the unique needs of diverse populations.

6. Collaboration and Teamwork: Ability to collaborate with other healthcare professionals and community stakeholders to develop comprehensive wellness programs and initiatives.

7. Continuous Learning: Commitment to continuous learning and staying updated on the latest research, trends, and best practices in lifestyle and wellness nursing.

8. Empathy and Motivational Skills: Empathy, compassion, and strong motivational skills to inspire individuals to make positive lifestyle changes and maintain long-term wellness habits.

Miscellaneous Information You Should Know

To enter the field of Lifestyle and Wellness Nursing, consider the following:

1. Gain Relevant Experience: Seek opportunities to gain experience in health education, lifestyle counseling, or wellness coaching. This can be through internships, volunteer work, or clinical rotations in settings that focus on lifestyle and wellness promotion.

2. Obtain Additional Certifications: Consider obtaining certifications in health coaching, nutrition counseling, or other related areas to enhance knowledge and demonstrate specialized expertise.

3. Networking: Connect with professionals working in lifestyle and wellness programs, health promotion departments, or community organizations to gain insights, mentorship, and potential job opportunities.

4. Pursue Continuing Education: Stay updated on the latest research, evidence-based interventions, and best practices in lifestyle and wellness nursing through continuing education, workshops, conferences, and professional development activities.

5. Specialty Organizations: Consider joining professional organizations related to lifestyle and wellness nursing, such as the American Holistic Nurses Association (AHNA) or the National Society of Health Coaches (NSHC), to connect with like-minded professionals and access valuable resources and networking opportunities.

Lifestyle and Wellness Nursing focuses on empowering individuals and communities to make positive lifestyle changes that promote health and well-being. By providing education, counseling, and ongoing support, Lifestyle, and Wellness Nurses play a crucial role in helping individuals achieve their wellness goals and improve their overall quality of life.

| Developmental Disabilities Nursing |

Developmental disabilities nursing involves providing specialized care to individuals with developmental disabilities, such as intellectual disabilities, autism spectrum disorder, Down syndrome, or cerebral palsy. Developmental disabilities nurses support individuals across the lifespan and focus on promoting their health, independence, and quality of life. They assess individual needs, develop care plans, administer treatments, provide education, and coordinate with interdisciplinary teams and community resources.

A Day in the Life

A typical day in the life of a developmental disabilities nurse may involve:

1. Assessing and monitoring the health status of individuals with developmental disabilities, including physical, cognitive, and behavioral assessments.
2. Administering medications and treatments as prescribed, including managing chronic conditions or addressing acute health concerns.
3. Developing and implementing individualized care plans based on the unique needs and goals of each individual.
4. Providing health education and support to individuals, their families, and caregivers regarding medication management, self-care, and promoting overall well-being.
5. Collaborating with interdisciplinary teams, such as physicians, therapists, social workers, and educators, to ensure comprehensive care and individualized treatment plans.
6. Advocating for individuals with developmental disabilities, ensuring their rights, needs, and preferences are respected and addressed.
7. Coordinating and accessing community resources, support services, and specialized therapies to enhance individuals' quality of life.
8. Maintaining accurate documentation and records related to health assessments, care plans, and interventions.
9. Staying updated on current research, evidence-based practices, and emerging therapies in the field of developmental disabilities nursing.

Degree(s) Required

To become a developmental disabilities nurse, you need to earn a degree in nursing. The two common degree paths are an Associate Degree in Nursing (ADN) or a Bachelor of Science in Nursing (BSN). However, pursuing a BSN is increasingly preferred for this specialty due to the comprehensive knowledge and critical thinking skills gained. Additionally, obtaining a Master of Science in Nursing (MSN) or a Doctor of Nursing Practice (DNP) can provide advanced training and leadership opportunities in developmental disabilities nursing.

Salary
$60,080 - $99,840

Specialty Certifications Available or Needed
Certification in developmental disabilities nursing can demonstrate specialized knowledge and expertise. The Developmental Disabilities Nurses Association (DDNA) offers the Developmental Disabilities Nurse Certification (DDNC) credential. Eligibility for the DDNC certification typically requires a combination of education, clinical experience, and the successful completion of an exam.

Job Requirements
Developmental disabilities nursing requires strong clinical skills, empathy, patience, and the ability to work effectively with individuals with diverse needs and communication styles. Job requirements may include:

1. Proficiency in assessing and managing common health conditions and complications associated with developmental disabilities.
2. Knowledge of developmental milestones, behavioral management techniques, and specialized therapies.
3. Ability to develop individualized care plans, considering the unique needs and goals of each individual.
4. Competence in providing health education, promoting self-care, and supporting individuals with developmental disabilities in achieving optimal health outcomes.
5. Effective communication skills to interact with individuals, families, caregivers, and interdisciplinary teams.
6. Advocacy skills to ensure individuals' rights, preferences, and needs are respected and addressed within the healthcare system.
7. Cultural competence to provide culturally sensitive care to individuals from diverse backgrounds.

Miscellaneous Information You Should Know
To enter the developmental disabilities nursing specialty, you may consider the following:

1. Gain experience in developmental disabilities settings: Acquiring experience in settings that serve individuals with developmental disabilities, such as developmental centers, group homes, schools, or clinics, can

provide a foundation for developmental disabilities nursing. Seek opportunities to work directly with individuals with developmental disabilities to develop knowledge and skills specific to this population.

2. Pursue additional education or certifications: Consider pursuing additional education or certifications specific to developmental disabilities nursing. This may include continuing education courses, workshops, or certificate programs focused on developmental disabilities. These opportunities can enhance your expertise and demonstrate your commitment to the specialty.

3. Develop effective communication skills: Communication is key in working with individuals with developmental disabilities. Enhance your communication skills to effectively engage and interact with individuals, their families, and caregivers. Learn strategies to adapt communication styles to the specific needs and abilities of individuals with developmental disabilities.

4. Cultural competence and sensitivity: Developmental disabilities nursing involves caring for individuals from diverse backgrounds. Develop cultural competence to provide respectful and individualized care that considers cultural beliefs, values, and practices.

5. Networking and professional involvement: Engage with professional organizations like the Developmental Disabilities Nurses Association (DDNA) to connect with other professionals in the field. Networking can provide opportunities for mentorship, collaboration, and staying informed about job opportunities or emerging practices.

Remember that specific requirements and preferences may vary depending on the healthcare organization, geographical location, and level of experience desired for developmental disabilities nursing positions.

| Home Health Nursing |

Home health nursing is a specialized field that focuses on providing healthcare services to patients in their own homes. Home health nurses work with patients of all ages who require skilled nursing care or assistance with activities of daily living. They play a vital role in assessing patients' needs, developing care plans, providing treatments, and educating patients and their families on managing their health conditions at home.

A Day in the Life
A typical day in the life of a home health nurse may involve:

1. Reviewing patient cases, assessing their needs, and planning visits based on patients' conditions and care requirements.
2. Traveling to patients' homes and performing comprehensive assessments, including physical, psychosocial, and environmental evaluations.
3. Administering medications, providing wound care, managing catheters, and performing other skilled nursing procedures as needed.
4. Monitoring patients' vital signs, observing any changes in their condition, and communicating updates to the healthcare team.
5. Collaborating with physicians, therapists, social workers, and other healthcare professionals involved in the patient's care to ensure coordinated and comprehensive services.
6. Educating patients and their families on disease management, medication administration, symptom recognition, and self-care techniques.
7. Assessing the safety of the home environment and providing recommendations for modifications or adaptations to promote patient well-being.
8. Documenting patient assessments, interventions, and responses accurately and maintaining proper records.
9. Participating in case conferences or team meetings to discuss patient progress, update care plans, and coordinate care transitions.
10. Engaging in ongoing professional development and staying updated on the latest home health practices and regulations.

Degree(s) Required
To become a home health nurse, you need to earn a degree in nursing. The two common degree paths are an Associate Degree in Nursing (ADN) or a Bachelor of Science in Nursing (BSN). However, some employers may prefer or require a BSN for home health nursing positions due to the comprehensive knowledge and critical thinking skills gained.

Salary
$64,370 - $103,140

Specialty Certifications Available or Needed
Certification in home health nursing can demonstrate specialized knowledge and competence. The Home Care Certification (HCC) is offered by the American Nurses Credentialing Center (ANCC) for nurses working in home health. Eligibility for the HCC certification typically requires a combination of education, clinical experience, and the successful completion of an exam.

Job Requirements
Home health nursing requires a strong foundation in medical-surgical nursing skills, as well as additional knowledge and skills specific to providing care in a home setting. Job requirements may include:

1. Proficiency in assessing and managing patients with various health conditions in a home environment, including monitoring vital signs, identifying complications, and recognizing changes in health status.

2. Knowledge of common chronic diseases, such as diabetes, heart disease, respiratory disorders, or neurological conditions, and their management in a home care setting.

3. Competence in performing skilled nursing procedures, such as wound care, intravenous therapy, medication administration, or catheter management, while ensuring patient safety and infection control.

4. Skill in developing individualized care plans that address patients' needs, goals, and preferences, while considering the home environment and available resources.

5. Effective communication skills to educate patients and their families, facilitate shared decision-making, and coordinate care with the healthcare team.

6. Understanding of community resources, social services, and support systems available to assist patients in their home care.

7. Proficiency in documentation and record-keeping, ensuring accurate and complete documentation of patient assessments, care plans, and interventions.

Miscellaneous Information You Should Know
To enter the home health nursing specialty, you may consider the following:

1. Gain clinical experience in relevant areas: Acquire experience in

medical-surgical units, community health settings, or home healthcare agencies to develop a foundation in assessing and managing patients with various health conditions and providing care in non-hospital settings.

2. Develop time management and organizational skills: Home health nursing often involves managing a caseload of patients with diverse needs. Enhance your ability to prioritize tasks, plan visits efficiently, and ensure continuity of care.

3. Familiarize yourself with regulations and policies: Gain knowledge of regulatory requirements, reimbursement guidelines, and documentation standards specific to home health nursing. Stay updated on changes in regulations and policies that may impact home healthcare practices.

4. Develop effective communication and patient education skills: Effective communication is crucial in home health nursing to establish trust, facilitate patient education, and ensure compliance with care plans. Enhance your ability to adapt your communication style to patients' and families' needs and cultural backgrounds.

5. Stay updated with evidence-based practices: Keep yourself informed about current research, evidence-based practices, and clinical guidelines related to home health nursing. Access resources provided by professional organizations, such as the Home Healthcare Nurses Association (HHNA), to stay up-to-date with emerging practices and advancements in the field.

6. Networking and professional involvement: Engage with professional organizations and attend conferences or seminars related to home health nursing. Connect with other home health nurses, access educational resources, and stay informed about career opportunities in the field.

Remember that specific requirements and preferences may vary depending on the healthcare organization, geographical location, and level of experience desired for home health nursing positions.

| Military Nursing |

Military nursing is a specialized field that involves providing healthcare services to active-duty military personnel, veterans, and their families. Military nurses serve in various branches of the military, including the Army, Navy, Air Force, and Coast Guard. They work in military hospitals, clinics, field medical units, or on military bases, and they play a critical role in maintaining the health and well-being of military personnel during peacetime and in times of conflict or humanitarian missions.

A Day in the Life

A typical day in the life of a military nurse may involve:

1. Providing direct patient care to military personnel, including conducting assessments, administering medications, and performing treatments as needed.

2. Assisting with medical evaluations and pre-deployment health screenings to ensure the fitness and readiness of military personnel for their assigned duties.

3. Collaborating with the healthcare team, including physicians, surgeons, and other military healthcare professionals, to provide comprehensive and coordinated care.

4. Participating in military exercises, field training, or deployments to support healthcare services in various operational environments.

5. Assisting with emergency medical care and trauma management in combat or disaster situations.

6. Educating military personnel on preventive health measures, health promotion, and wellness strategies.

7. Managing and organizing medical supplies, equipment, and medications to ensure readiness and availability in military healthcare settings.

8. Assisting with research and evidence-based practice initiatives to improve military healthcare delivery and outcomes.

9. Providing support and counseling to military personnel and their families, addressing the unique challenges and stresses associated with military life.

10. Engaging in ongoing military training and professional development to maintain readiness and stay updated on the latest advancements in military nursing practices.

Degree(s) Required

To become a military nurse, you need to earn a degree in nursing. The two common degree paths are an Associate Degree in Nursing (ADN) or a Bachelor of Science in Nursing (BSN). However, some branches of the military may prefer or require a BSN for military nursing positions due to the comprehensive knowledge and critical thinking skills gained.

Salary
$65,000 - $107,500 *(most often dictated by rank)*

Specialty Certifications Available or Needed
While there isn't a specific certification dedicated solely to military nursing, specialized certifications in areas such as critical care, emergency nursing, or trauma nursing can be valuable in a military nursing career. These certifications demonstrate advanced knowledge and competence in specific areas of practice and may enhance career opportunities within the military healthcare system.

Job Requirements
Military nursing requires a strong foundation in nursing practice, as well as additional knowledge and skills related to military healthcare, emergency care, and operational medicine. Job requirements may include:

1. Proficiency in providing direct patient care and emergency medical services in a military healthcare setting.
2. Knowledge of military healthcare policies, regulations, and guidelines related to medical readiness, deployment health, and healthcare delivery in austere environments.
3. Understanding of military operational medicine, including triage, combat casualty care, and trauma management.
4. Competence in working within the military chain of command, following military protocols, and adhering to military standards of professionalism and conduct.
5. Effective communication and leadership skills to work collaboratively with military personnel, other healthcare professionals, and diverse populations.
6. Ability to adapt to changing environments, work in high-stress situations, and make critical decisions quickly and efficiently.
7. Proficiency in documentation and record-keeping, ensuring accurate and complete documentation of patient assessments, treatments, and responses.
8. Collaboration with the military healthcare team, including physicians, surgeons, medics, and other military healthcare professionals, to provide coordinated and mission-focused care.
9. Flexibility and willingness to serve in various military healthcare settings, including deployed environments or remote locations.

10. Meeting the physical and medical requirements set by the military branch, which may include passing physical fitness tests and meeting specific health standards.

Miscellaneous Information You Should Know

To enter the military nursing specialty, you may consider the following:

1. Joining the military as a nurse: Research the requirements and opportunities within each branch of the military (Army, Navy, Air Force, Coast Guard) and consider applying to the specific branch that aligns with your career goals and interests. Each branch has its own recruitment process and specific criteria for accepting nurses into their ranks.

2. Meeting military enlistment criteria: Ensure that you meet the basic eligibility criteria for military service, which may include age restrictions, citizenship requirements, physical fitness standards, and medical clearance.

3. Developing leadership and teamwork skills: Engage in activities that foster leadership, teamwork, and adaptability, as these skills are highly valued in military nursing.

4. Stay updated with military healthcare practices: Keep yourself informed about military healthcare policies, regulations, and practices. Access resources provided by military healthcare organizations, attend military healthcare conferences or workshops, and engage with military nursing communities to stay up-to-date with the latest developments in military healthcare.

5. Prepare for military-specific training: Understand that military nursing may involve additional training, such as Basic Officer Leadership Courses (BOLC), Military Combat Casualty Care (MC3), or other military-specific courses, depending on the branch of service.

Remember that specific requirements and preferences may vary depending on the military branch, geographical location, and specific roles within military nursing. It's important to consult with a recruiter or military healthcare representative to obtain accurate and up-to-date information about the requirements and opportunities in military nursing.

| School Nursing |

School nursing is a specialized field of nursing that focuses on promoting the health and well-being of students in educational settings. School nurses play a crucial role in providing direct healthcare services, managing chronic conditions, promoting health education, and ensuring a safe and healthy environment for students. They collaborate with students, parents, teachers, and other healthcare professionals to address health needs and support students' academic success.

A Day in the Life

A typical day in the life of a school nurse may involve:

1. Health Assessments: Conducting health assessments of students, including screenings for vision, hearing, and other health conditions. Assessing and addressing acute illnesses, injuries, and chronic health conditions.

2. Medication Management: Administering prescribed medications to students, monitoring medication compliance, and maintaining medication records. Providing education to students and staff regarding medication administration and management.

3. First Aid and Emergency Care: Providing first aid and emergency care to students who experience injuries, accidents, or sudden illnesses. Collaborating with emergency response personnel as necessary.

4. Chronic Disease Management: Managing chronic health conditions in students, such as asthma, diabetes, allergies, and epilepsy. Developing and implementing individualized healthcare plans (IHPs) to ensure students' safety and appropriate management of their conditions.

5. Health Promotion and Education: Developing and delivering health promotion programs, including presentations, workshops, and educational materials on topics like nutrition, hygiene, mental health, and sexual health. Collaborating with teachers and staff to integrate health education into the school curriculum.

6. Immunization Compliance: Ensuring students' compliance with immunization requirements and maintaining immunization records. Collaborating with public health authorities to track and manage communicable diseases.

7. Health Counseling: Providing health counseling to students, addressing concerns related to physical, mental, and emotional well-being. Referring students to appropriate healthcare providers or community resources when necessary.

8. Health Screenings and Referrals: Conducting screenings for conditions such as scoliosis, obesity, and mental health concerns. Referring

students for further evaluation or treatment as needed.

9. Collaboration with the School Community: Collaborating with teachers, administrators, and other school personnel to create a safe and healthy environment. Participating in school safety committees and supporting emergency preparedness plans.

10. Documentation and Record-Keeping: Maintaining accurate and confidential health records for students, including health assessments, immunization records, medication administration records, and incident reports.

Degree(s) Required

To become a school nurse, you need to earn a degree in nursing. The two common degree paths are an Associate Degree in Nursing (ADN) or a Bachelor of Science in Nursing (BSN). However, some school districts or states may require or prefer a BSN for school nursing positions due to the comprehensive knowledge and critical thinking skills gained.

Salary
$63,070 - $103,860

Specialty Certifications Available or Needed

Certification in school nursing can demonstrate specialized knowledge and competence. The National Board for Certification of School Nurses (NBCSN) offers the Certified School Nurse (CSN) credential. Eligibility for the CSN certification typically requires a combination of education, clinical experience in school nursing, and successful completion of an exam.

Job Requirements

School nursing requires a strong foundation in nursing practice, as well as additional knowledge and skills specific to the school setting. Job requirements may include:

1. Knowledge of child and adolescent health issues, growth, and development.

2. Familiarity with common acute and chronic health conditions in school-aged children, such as allergies, asthma, diabetes, and mental health concerns.

3. Competence in providing first aid, emergency care, and managing health-related emergencies.

4. Understanding of immunization requirements, communicable disease control, and public health practices relevant to schools.

5. Collaboration and communication skills to work effectively with

students, parents, teachers, administrators, and other healthcare professionals.

6. Ability to assess and manage acute illnesses and injuries, as well as develop and implement healthcare plans for students with chronic conditions.

7. Knowledge of health promotion strategies, including developing and delivering age-appropriate health education programs.

8. Documentation and record-keeping skills to maintain accurate and confidential health records for students.

9. Ability to navigate and comply with state and federal regulations, as well as school policies related to health services in educational settings.

10. Strong communication and advocacy skills to address health concerns and promote the well-being of students.

Miscellaneous Information You Should Know

To enter the school nursing specialty, you may consider the following:

1. Gain clinical experience with pediatric populations: Seek opportunities to gain clinical experience working with children and adolescents in various healthcare settings, such as pediatric clinics, hospitals, or community health centers. This experience will provide valuable exposure to the unique healthcare needs of school-aged children.

2. Pursue additional education or certifications in school nursing: While certification in school nursing is not mandatory in all jurisdictions, it can enhance your knowledge and marketability. Consider pursuing certifications such as the Certified School Nurse (CSN) offered by the National Board for Certification of School Nurses (NBCSN).

3. Understand state and local regulations: Familiarize yourself with the specific requirements and regulations for school nursing in your state or region. This may include obtaining the necessary licensure or endorsement specific to school nursing.

4. Networking and professional involvement: Engage with professional organizations, such as the National Association of School Nurses (NASN), to connect with other school nurses, access educational resources, and stay informed about career opportunities. Participate in conferences, webinars, or local chapter meetings to expand your knowledge and network with professionals in the field.

Remember that specific requirements and preferences may vary depending on the school district, state regulations, and level of experience desired for school nursing positions.

| Disaster Nursing |

Disaster Nursing is a specialized field that focuses on providing emergency medical care and support during and after disasters and emergencies. Disaster Nurses play a crucial role in managing the health and safety of individuals affected by natural disasters, pandemics, terrorist attacks, and other emergencies. They are trained to assess, triage, and provide immediate medical assistance to those in need, as well as coordinate with other healthcare professionals and emergency response teams to ensure effective disaster response and recovery.

A Day in the Life

A typical day in the life of a Disaster Nurse may involve:

1. Preparedness and Planning: Participating in disaster preparedness activities, such as creating emergency response plans, conducting drills and simulations, and collaborating with local emergency management agencies.

2. Emergency Response: Mobilizing to the disaster site or designated medical facilities to provide immediate medical care to victims, including triaging patients, performing emergency medical procedures, administering first aid, and stabilizing critical patients.

3. Triage and Prioritization: Assessing and categorizing patients based on the severity of their injuries or illnesses to ensure that those with life-threatening conditions receive immediate attention and appropriate resources are allocated effectively.

4. Medical Treatment and Care: Administering medications, providing wound care, managing pain, and addressing acute and chronic health conditions in a high-stress environment with limited resources.

5. Collaborative Care: Working closely with other healthcare professionals, such as physicians, nurses, paramedics, and social workers, to deliver comprehensive care and ensure continuity of care during the disaster response.

6. Public Health Measures: Implementing public health measures to prevent the spread of infectious diseases, including administering vaccinations, promoting hygiene practices, and providing health education to affected individuals and communities.

7. Psychological Support: Providing emotional support and counseling to survivors and their families, addressing psychological trauma, grief, and post-disaster stress.

8. Resource Management: Managing and coordinating medical supplies, equipment, and personnel to ensure efficient utilization of resources and meet the changing needs of the disaster situation.

9. Documentation and Reporting: Maintaining accurate and detailed records of patient assessments, treatments, and interventions, as well as participating in data collection for epidemiological purposes and quality improvement initiatives.

10. Disaster Recovery: Participating in post-disaster recovery efforts, including providing ongoing healthcare services, collaborating with community organizations, and assisting in the rebuilding and restoration of healthcare infrastructure.

11. Continuous Education: Engaging in ongoing training and education related to disaster response, emergency management, disaster nursing protocols, and public health principles.

Degree(s) Required

To pursue a career in Disaster Nursing, a minimum of an Associate Degree in Nursing (ADN) or a Bachelor of Science in Nursing (BSN) is typically required. However, some employers may prefer or require a BSN due to the complex and specialized nature of disaster nursing. Additionally, obtaining an advanced degree in nursing, such as a Master of Science in Nursing (MSN) or Doctor of Nursing Practice (DNP), can provide advanced knowledge and leadership opportunities in disaster nursing.

Salary
$68,450 - $115,800

Specialty Certifications Available or Needed

While there isn't a specific certification exclusively for Disaster Nursing, there are certifications that can enhance your skills and knowledge in emergency and critical care situations, which are highly relevant to the field of disaster nursing. These certifications may include:

1. Emergency Nurse Certification (CEN): Offered by the Board of Certification for Emergency Nursing (BCEN), the CEN certification validates your expertise in emergency nursing and demonstrates your ability to provide competent care in emergency situations.

2. Trauma Certified Registered Nurse (TCRN): The TCRN certification, offered by the Board of Certification for Emergency Nursing (BCEN), focuses on trauma nursing and is relevant in disaster situations where trauma care is required.

3. Critical Care Registered Nurse (CCRN): The CCRN certification, offered by the American Association of Critical-Care Nurses (AACN), validates your specialized knowledge and skills in critical care nursing, which are highly relevant in disaster response and management.

While not specific to disaster nursing, these certifications can enhance your competence in providing emergency and critical care in high-pressure situations.

Job Requirements

To work as a Disaster Nurse, consider the following job requirements:

1. Emergency and Critical Care Skills: Strong clinical skills in emergency and critical care, including rapid assessment, triage, wound care, emergency procedures, and the ability to make quick and effective decisions under pressure.
2. Disaster Management Knowledge: Understanding of disaster management principles, emergency response protocols, incident command systems, and public health measures related to disaster preparedness, response, and recovery.
3. Interdisciplinary Collaboration: Ability to collaborate effectively with multidisciplinary teams, including emergency management personnel, public health officials, law enforcement agencies, and community organizations.
4. Flexibility and Adaptability: Capacity to adapt to rapidly changing situations, work in resource-constrained environments, and manage high-stress and emotionally challenging circumstances.
5. Effective Communication: Strong communication and interpersonal skills to effectively communicate with patients, families, healthcare team members, and community stakeholders during emergencies.
6. Cultural Competence: Sensitivity and awareness of cultural diversity to provide patient-centered care and respect the unique needs and beliefs of individuals and communities affected by disasters.
7. Leadership and Decision-Making: Leadership qualities, critical thinking skills, and the ability to make sound decisions in high-pressure situations while prioritizing patient needs and allocating resources appropriately.
8. Disaster Nursing Training: Completion of specialized training programs, workshops, or certifications related to disaster nursing, emergency management, incident command systems, or public health emergency response can be beneficial.

Miscellaneous Information You Should Know

To enter the field of Disaster Nursing, consider the following:

1. Gain Experience in Emergency and Critical Care: Acquiring

experience in emergency departments, critical care units, or trauma centers can provide you with the necessary skills and exposure to high-stress healthcare environments.

2. Volunteer or Intern: Seek opportunities to volunteer or intern with organizations involved in disaster response and recovery, such as the Red Cross or local emergency management agencies.

3. Pursue Additional Education: Consider pursuing advanced education or training programs in emergency management, disaster nursing, or public health emergency response to deepen your knowledge and expertise in the field.

4. Professional Organizations: Joining professional organizations, such as the Emergency Nurses Association (ENA) or the International Council of Nurses (ICN), can provide networking opportunities, access to resources, and professional development in disaster nursing.

Entering the field of Disaster Nursing offers an opportunity to make a significant impact during emergencies and disasters by providing immediate medical care, support, and coordination to those affected. It requires resilience, adaptability, and a commitment to lifelong learning in order to effectively respond to the complex challenges posed by disasters and emergencies.

| Faith Community Nursing |

Faith Community Nursing, also known as Parish Nursing or Congregational Nursing, is a specialized field that combines spiritual care and health promotion within a faith community. Faith Community Nurses serve as a bridge between healthcare and faith, providing holistic care that integrates the physical, emotional, and spiritual well-being of individuals and communities. They work within religious organizations to promote health education, provide support to individuals and families, advocate for health-related issues, and facilitate access to healthcare resources.

A Day in the Life

A typical day in the life of a Faith Community Nurse may involve:

1. Health Education and Promotion: Conducting health education sessions and workshops within the faith community on topics such as preventive care, healthy lifestyles, chronic disease management, mental health, and spiritual well-being.

2. Pastoral Care and Support: Offering spiritual care, prayer, and emotional support to individuals and families facing health challenges, loss, or other life transitions.

3. Health Screenings and Assessments: Conducting health screenings, assessments, and risk factor evaluations within the faith community to identify potential health issues and provide appropriate referrals or interventions.

4. Referrals and Resource Coordination: Assisting individuals and families in navigating the healthcare system by providing information about available resources, connecting them with healthcare providers, and facilitating access to healthcare services.

5. Care Coordination and Case Management: Collaborating with healthcare professionals, community agencies, and social services to coordinate care and support for individuals with complex health needs.

6. Advocacy: Advocating for the health needs and concerns of the faith community, addressing health disparities, promoting health policy changes, and organizing community health initiatives.

7. Spiritual Support: Providing spiritual guidance, counseling, and bereavement support to individuals and families during times of illness, loss, and spiritual distress.

8. Collaboration with Faith Leaders: Collaborating with faith leaders and clergy to integrate health and wellness into religious services, incorporating health-related prayers, rituals, and support into the faith community's activities.

9. Crisis Response: Assisting the faith community during times of

crisis or emergencies, providing support and coordinating resources for affected individuals and families.

10. Health Counseling: Offering one-on-one health counseling to address individual health concerns, promote healthy behaviors, and develop care plans tailored to individuals' specific needs.

11. Documentation and Reporting: Maintaining accurate and confidential records of interactions, assessments, referrals, and interventions in compliance with ethical and legal guidelines.

Degree(s) Required

To pursue a career in Faith Community Nursing, a minimum of an Associate Degree in Nursing (ADN) or a Bachelor of Science in Nursing (BSN) is typically required. However, some faith communities and employers may prefer or require a BSN due to the specialized nature of faith community nursing. Additionally, obtaining an advanced degree in nursing, such as a Master of Science in Nursing (MSN), can provide advanced knowledge in spiritual care, community health, and leadership.

Salary
$63,070 - $103,680

Specialty Certifications Available or Needed

While there isn't a specific certification exclusively for Faith Community Nursing, there are certifications and training programs available that can enhance your knowledge and skills in spiritual care and community health. Some relevant certifications include:

1. Faith Community Nurse Certification: Offered by the Westberg Institute for Faith Community Nursing, this certification validates the knowledge and competencies of Faith Community Nurses and provides recognition in the field.

2. Advanced Practice Hospice and Palliative Care Nursing Certification: This certification, offered by various organizations, focuses on providing expert care for individuals with advanced illness and addressing their physical, emotional, and spiritual needs.

While not specific to Faith Community Nursing, these certifications can enhance your expertise in areas related to spiritual care, end-of-life care, and holistic health.

Job Requirements

To work as a Faith Community Nurse, consider the following job requirements:

1. Spiritual and Cultural Sensitivity: Ability to respect and understand diverse religious beliefs, cultural practices, and values within the faith community.

2. Strong Communication Skills: Effective communication skills to interact with individuals, families, faith leaders, and healthcare professionals in a compassionate and culturally sensitive manner.

3. Knowledge of Health Promotion and Education: Understanding of health promotion principles, preventive care, and health education strategies to deliver comprehensive health messages to the faith community.

4. Collaboration and Teamwork: Ability to collaborate with faith leaders, clergy, healthcare professionals, community organizations, and volunteers to promote health and wellness within the faith community.

5. Ethical Considerations: Adherence to ethical guidelines and legal regulations regarding confidentiality, informed consent, and boundaries when providing spiritual and health-related care.

6. Flexibility and Adaptability: Ability to work in diverse settings and adapt to the needs and resources available within the faith community.

7. Ongoing Education and Professional Development: Engagement in continuing education, workshops, and conferences related to faith community nursing, spiritual care, health promotion, and community health.

Miscellaneous Information You Should Know

To enter the field of Faith Community Nursing, consider the following:

1. Gain Experience in Community Health: Acquiring experience in community health nursing or public health settings can provide valuable knowledge and skills in population-based care and community engagement.

2. Engage with Faith Communities: Seek opportunities to volunteer or engage with local faith communities to gain exposure to their health-related needs, values, and practices.

3. Obtain Spiritual Care Training: Seek additional training or certifications in spiritual care, pastoral counseling, or chaplaincy to deepen your understanding of the spiritual needs and practices within a faith community.

4. Professional Organizations: Join professional organizations, such as the Westberg Institute for Faith Community Nursing, to access resources, networking opportunities, and educational programs specific to faith community nursing.

*Working as a Faith Community Nurse allows you to integrate your nursing skills with *spiritual care, promoting health and well-being within a faith community. It requires a deep understanding and respect for diverse religious beliefs, cultural practices, and the ability to provide holistic care that addresses the physical, emotional, and spiritual needs of individuals and communities.*

| Correctional Nursing |

Correctional Nursing is a unique nursing specialty that focuses on providing healthcare services to individuals who are incarcerated in correctional facilities such as jails, prisons, and detention centers. Correctional Nurses work in collaboration with correctional officers and healthcare teams to deliver comprehensive care to a diverse patient population. They provide medical assessments, administer treatments and medications, manage chronic conditions, respond to emergencies, and promote health education and disease prevention within the correctional setting.

A Day in the Life
A typical day in the life of a Correctional Nurse may involve:

1. Patient Assessments: Conducting initial health assessments to evaluate patients' medical history, current health status, and healthcare needs. Assessing for acute and chronic conditions, mental health concerns, and substance abuse issues.

2. Medication Administration: Administering medications according to prescribed orders, ensuring accurate dosage, documentation, and proper medication management procedures. Following the facility's medication administration policies and guidelines.

3. Chronic Disease Management: Managing and monitoring chronic diseases such as diabetes, hypertension, asthma, and infectious diseases within the correctional population. Collaborating with healthcare teams to develop treatment plans, provide education, and promote self-care.

4. Emergency Response: Responding to medical emergencies, trauma situations, and mental health crises within the correctional facility. Assisting in resuscitation efforts, stabilizing patients, and coordinating transfers to higher levels of care if needed.

5. Health Education: Providing health education to inmates on various topics such as chronic disease management, medication adherence, healthy lifestyle choices, and preventive care. Conducting group education sessions and one-on-one counseling as needed.

6. Mental Health Support: Assessing and addressing the mental health needs of inmates, including evaluating for signs of depression, anxiety, or other mental health disorders. Collaborating with mental health professionals to provide appropriate interventions and referrals.

7. Collaboration with Multidisciplinary Team: Working closely with correctional officers, physicians, nurse practitioners, mental health professionals, and other healthcare staff to coordinate patient care, share information, and ensure comprehensive treatment plans.

8. Documentation and Reporting: Maintaining accurate and up-to-date medical records, documenting assessments, treatments, medications administered, and any incidents or encounters. Following facility protocols for documentation and reporting.

9. Safety and Security: Adhering to security measures within the correctional facility to maintain the safety and well-being of staff and patients. Following security protocols, maintaining awareness of potential risks, and maintaining personal safety.

10. Medication and Supply Management: Ensuring proper inventory management of medications, medical supplies, and equipment. Following facility policies for medication storage, security, and disposal.

11. Infection Control: Implementing infection control measures to prevent the spread of communicable diseases within the correctional facility. Educating inmates on hygiene practices and facilitating disease prevention strategies.

12. Crisis Intervention: Assisting in crisis intervention situations, de-escalating conflicts, and providing emotional support to inmates in distress. Collaborating with mental health professionals and correctional officers to maintain a safe environment.

13. Continuity of Care: Coordinating healthcare services and referrals for inmates upon their release from the correctional facility. Ensuring a smooth transition and facilitating access to community-based healthcare providers.

Degree(s) Required

To become a Correctional Nurse, you need to have a degree in nursing. The two common degree paths are an Associate Degree in Nursing (ADN) or a Bachelor of Science in Nursing (BSN). However, some employers may prefer or require a BSN due to the specialized nature of the role. Additionally, having a strong foundation in medical-surgical nursing, psychiatric nursing, and community health nursing is beneficial.

Salary
$64,470 - $107,740

Specialty Certifications Available or Needed

While not mandatory, obtaining specialty certifications related to correctional nursing can demonstrate your expertise and commitment to the field. One of the recognized certifications is:

1. Certified Correctional Health Professional (CCHP): Offered by the National Commission on Correctional Health Care (NCCHC), this certification validates your knowledge and skills in correctional healthcare.

It covers various areas such as clinical practice, security and administration, legal and ethical principles, and professional collaboration.

Obtaining the CCHP certification demonstrates your proficiency in providing healthcare within the correctional setting and adhering to the specific standards and guidelines.

Job Requirements

Correctional Nursing requires specific skills and qualities to provide quality care within the unique environment of correctional facilities. Job requirements may include:

1. Strong Assessment Skills: Proficiency in conducting comprehensive health assessments, including physical assessments, mental health assessments, and risk assessments.

2. Adaptability: Ability to adapt to the challenging and dynamic environment of a correctional facility, including managing unpredictable situations, working with diverse patient populations, and adhering to security protocols.

3. Communication Skills: Effective communication skills to interact with inmates, correctional officers, healthcare team members, and other stakeholders. Ability to communicate in a non-judgmental and culturally sensitive manner.

4. Knowledge of Correctional Systems: Understanding the policies, procedures, and regulations specific to the correctional environment. Familiarity with legal and ethical considerations in correctional healthcare.

5. Crisis Management Skills: Ability to respond calmly and effectively in crisis situations, including medical emergencies, mental health crises, and conflicts within the correctional facility.

6. Cultural Competence: Demonstrating cultural competence and sensitivity to work with diverse populations, respecting individual backgrounds, beliefs, and values.

7. Collaboration and Teamwork: Working collaboratively with multidisciplinary teams, including correctional officers, physicians, mental health professionals, and social workers, to provide comprehensive care and support.

8. Self-Care and Resilience: Recognizing the potential impact of working in a correctional environment and practicing self-care strategies to maintain physical and emotional well-being.

9. Licensing: Obtaining and maintaining a valid nursing license in the state where you practice. Complying with any additional licensing or credentialing requirements specific to correctional nursing set by your employer or local regulations.

Miscellaneous Information You Should Know

To enter the Correctional Nursing specialty, consider the following:

1. Gain Experience in Relevant Areas: Gaining experience in medical-surgical nursing, psychiatric nursing, community health, or public health can provide a foundation for working in the correctional setting. These areas often overlap with the healthcare needs of incarcerated individuals.

2. Familiarize Yourself with Correctional Systems: Acquiring knowledge about correctional systems, laws, and regulations can help you better understand the unique challenges and responsibilities of correctional nursing.

3. Training and Orientation: Employers typically provide specialized training and orientation programs for nurses entering the correctional setting. This may include education on security protocols, safety measures, and policies specific to the facility.

4. Continuing Education: Stay updated on the latest research, guidelines, and advancements in correctional nursing through continuing education opportunities. Attend workshops, conferences, or seminars specific to correctional healthcare.

5. Professional Networking: Engage with professional organizations and networks in the field of correctional nursing. Participate in meetings, connect with colleagues, and stay informed about new research and trends.

6. Personal Safety: Understand and adhere to the safety protocols and measures set by the correctional facility. Maintain personal safety by following security guidelines and being vigilant in your surroundings.

Entering the Correctional Nursing specialty requires a commitment to providing healthcare to an underserved population, the ability to work within a secure and challenging environment, and a dedication to promoting the health and well-being of incarcerated individuals.

| Government Nursing |

Government Nursing refers to nursing roles within government healthcare agencies, such as the Department of Health, public health departments, military health services, correctional facilities, and other government-funded healthcare institutions. Nurses working in government settings play a crucial role in providing healthcare services, implementing health policies, conducting health education and promotion, managing public health programs, and addressing the healthcare needs of diverse populations.

A Day in the Life

A typical day in the life of a Government Nurse may involve:

1. Health Services Delivery: Providing direct patient care, including assessments, treatments, administering medications, and performing procedures within the scope of practice.

2. Public Health Promotion: Conducting health education and promotion activities, including immunization programs, disease prevention initiatives, and health screenings.

3. Policy Implementation: Implementing and enforcing health policies and regulations, ensuring compliance with legal and ethical standards.

4. Epidemiology and Surveillance: Monitoring and investigating infectious diseases, outbreaks, and public health emergencies, and implementing appropriate control measures.

5. Collaboration and Coordination: Collaborating with interdisciplinary teams, community organizations, and government agencies to develop and implement public health programs and initiatives.

6. Data Collection and Analysis: Collecting and analyzing health data to assess population health, identify trends, and develop evidence-based interventions.

7. Research and Evaluation: Participating in research studies, conducting program evaluations, and contributing to evidence-based practices and policies.

8. Emergency Preparedness: Planning and responding to public health emergencies, such as natural disasters, epidemics, or bioterrorism incidents.

9. Health Policy Development: Contributing to the development and review of health policies, guidelines, and regulations at local, regional, or national levels.

10. Leadership and Management: Taking leadership roles in managing healthcare programs, overseeing budgets, and ensuring quality and safety standards are met.

Degree(s) Required

To pursue a career in Government Nursing, a minimum of a Bachelor of Science in Nursing (BSN) degree is typically required. However, higher-level degrees such as a Master of Science in Nursing (MSN) or Doctor of Nursing Practice (DNP) can provide advanced knowledge and skills in nursing leadership, policy, and healthcare management, which are valuable in government nursing roles.

Salary

$61,700 - $91,830

Specialty Certifications Available or Needed

While specific certifications may not be required for all government nursing positions, obtaining relevant certifications can enhance your knowledge and expertise in specific areas. Examples include:

1. Public Health Nurse (PHN): Certifications such as Certified Public Health Nurse (CPHN) or Advanced Public Health Nurse (APHN-BC) validate expertise in public health nursing.

2. Infection Control: Certifications such as the Certification in Infection Prevention and Control (CIC) or the Certified in Healthcare Quality and Management (CHCQM) with a focus on infection prevention and control demonstrate expertise in preventing and managing infectious diseases.

3. Emergency Preparedness: Certifications like the Certified Emergency Nurse (CEN) or the Certified Healthcare Emergency Professional (CHEP) provide specialized knowledge in emergency preparedness and response.

It's important to note that certification requirements may vary depending on the specific role and organization within government nursing.

Job Requirements

To work in Government Nursing, consider the following job requirements:

1. Licensure: Obtain a valid registered nursing license in the jurisdiction where you intend to work, meeting the requirements set by the nursing regulatory body.
2. Knowledge of Government Healthcare Systems: Understand the

structure, policies, and regulations of the specific government healthcare system where you seek employment.

3. Public Health Knowledge: Familiarize yourself with public health principles, epidemiology, health promotion, disease prevention, and health policy.

4. Communication and Collaboration: Possess strong communication, interpersonal, and teamwork skills to collaborate with diverse stakeholders, including government officials, colleagues, and community members.

5. Flexibility and Adaptability: Be adaptable to changing healthcare priorities, policies, and resource availability in government settings.

6. Leadership and Management: Demonstrate leadership skills, including the ability to lead teams, manage healthcare programs, and contribute to policy development.

7. Ethical and Legal Understanding: Comply with ethical standards, confidentiality requirements, and legal frameworks governing healthcare delivery and public health practice.

8. Knowledge of Health Data and Technology: Familiarize yourself with health information systems, data collection methods, and technology used in government healthcare settings.

9. Commitment to Public Service: Embrace the mission of serving the public, addressing health disparities, and promoting health equity.

10. Continuing Education: Stay updated with advances in nursing practice, public health, and healthcare policies through continuing education, conferences, and professional development activities.

Miscellaneous Information You Should Know

To enter the field of Government Nursing, consider the following:

1. Gain Experience in Public Health or Government Settings: Seek opportunities to gain experience in public health programs, government healthcare agencies, or community health initiatives to familiarize yourself with the unique aspects of government nursing.

2. Networking and Professional Engagement: Join professional organizations related to government nursing, such as the American Nurses Association (ANA), the Association of Public Health Nurses (APHN), or specialty-specific organizations, to network with professionals in the field and access resources.

3. Consider Advanced Education: Pursuing a Master's degree or specialized training in public health, healthcare administration, or health policy can enhance your knowledge and open up opportunities for leadership roles within government nursing.

Working in Government Nursing offers diverse opportunities to make a significant impact on public health, shape health policies, and improve healthcare delivery within a government setting. It requires a solid understanding of public health principles, effective communication and collaboration skills, and the ability to adapt to evolving healthcare policies and priorities.

| Camp Nursing |

Camp Nursing is a specialized field of nursing that focuses on providing healthcare services to individuals at camps, including summer camps, wilderness camps, and recreational camps. Camp Nurses play a crucial role in ensuring the health and safety of campers and staff members. They provide both routine and emergency medical care, manage chronic health conditions, administer medications, and promote a healthy camp environment.

A Day in the Life

A typical day in the life of a Camp Nurse may involve:

1. Health Assessments: Conducting health assessments upon arrival to evaluate the overall health status of campers and staff members. Assessing for any pre-existing medical conditions, allergies, medications, and immunization status.

2. Medication Administration: Administering routine medications to campers with chronic health conditions, such as asthma, diabetes, or allergies. Ensuring proper medication management, dosage administration, and maintaining medication records.

3. First Aid and Emergency Care: Providing first aid and immediate care for injuries, illnesses, and emergencies that may occur at the camp. This includes assessing and treating minor injuries, managing acute illnesses, and coordinating emergency medical services when necessary.

4. Health Education: Conducting health education sessions and promoting health and safety practices among campers and staff. Topics may include personal hygiene, sun protection, hydration, insect bite prevention, and basic first aid.

5. Health Records and Documentation: Maintaining accurate and up-to-date health records for each camper and staff member. Documenting all health assessments, treatments, medications administered, and any incidents or emergencies that occur.

6. Illness and Infection Control: Monitoring and managing communicable diseases or outbreaks that may occur within the camp setting. Implementing infection control measures, such as isolation protocols and hygiene practices, to prevent the spread of illnesses.

7. Collaborative Care: Collaborating with camp directors, counselors, and other camp staff to ensure the overall well-being and safety of campers. Communicating and coordinating with parents or guardians regarding health concerns, medication management, and treatment plans.

8. Health Promotion: Promoting healthy lifestyle choices and recreational activities to enhance the campers' physical and mental well-

being. Encouraging physical activity, proper nutrition, and adequate rest.

9. Preparedness and Emergency Planning: Participating in camp safety drills and emergency preparedness activities. Assisting in developing emergency response plans and protocols specific to the camp setting.

10. Adherence to Regulatory Standards: Complying with applicable state and local regulations, licensing requirements, and healthcare standards related to camp nursing. Staying updated on current best practices and guidelines in camp healthcare.

Degree(s) Required

To become a Camp Nurse, you need to have a degree in nursing. The two common degree paths are an Associate Degree in Nursing (ADN) or a Bachelor of Science in Nursing (BSN). However, specific requirements may vary depending on the camp's regulations and the level of responsibility involved.

Salary
$63,070 - $103,680

Specialty Certifications Available or Needed

While there are no specific certifications exclusively for Camp Nursing, obtaining certifications related to pediatric nursing or emergency nursing can be beneficial. Examples of relevant certifications include:

1. Pediatric Nursing Certification (CPN): Offered by the Pediatric Nursing Certification Board (PNCB), this certification validates expertise in pediatric nursing and demonstrates specialized knowledge in caring for children and adolescents.

2. Emergency Nursing Certification (CEN): Offered by the Board of Certification for Emergency Nursing (BCEN), this certification demonstrates proficiency in emergency nursing practice and knowledge in emergency care management.

While not mandatory, these certifications can enhance your knowledge and credibility as a Camp Nurse.

Job Requirements

Camp Nursing requires specific skills and qualities to ensure the health and safety of campers. Job requirements may include:

1. Pediatric Care Skills: Proficiency in providing care to children and adolescents, including assessment, medication administration, and

treatment of common pediatric conditions.

2. Emergency Response Skills: Ability to recognize and manage common injuries and illnesses that may occur in the camp setting, including first aid, basic life support (BLS), and the ability to coordinate emergency medical services.

3. Communication and Interpersonal Skills: Effective communication skills to interact with campers, parents, camp staff, and healthcare professionals. Ability to provide clear instructions, listen attentively, and display empathy and compassion.

4. Organization and Adaptability: Strong organizational skills to manage multiple tasks, prioritize care needs, and respond to changing situations in a fast-paced camp environment.

5. Collaboration and Teamwork: Ability to work collaboratively with camp staff, counselors, and other healthcare professionals to ensure coordinated and holistic care for campers.

6. Cultural Sensitivity: Respect for cultural diversity and the ability to provide culturally competent care to campers from diverse backgrounds.

7. Physical and Mental Stamina: Camp Nursing may require long hours, physical stamina, and the ability to handle stressful situations with resilience.

8. Licensing and Credentialing: Obtaining and maintaining a valid nursing license in the state where the camp is located. Complying with any additional licensing or credentialing requirements specific to camp nursing set by the camp or local regulations.

Miscellaneous Information You Should Know

To enter the Camp Nursing specialty, consider the following:

1. Experience with Pediatrics: Gaining experience in pediatric nursing, either through clinical rotations or employment, can provide a strong foundation for camp nursing. Familiarize yourself with common pediatric conditions, medication dosages, and age-appropriate care.

2. First Aid and CPR Certification: Acquiring certification in first aid and cardiopulmonary resuscitation (CPR) is typically required for camp nursing positions. These certifications demonstrate your ability to respond to emergencies and provide initial care.

3. Camp Nurse Training: Many camps provide specific training programs for their nurses, which may cover topics such as camp health policies, emergency response protocols, and camp-specific procedures. Familiarize yourself with these training requirements and be prepared to participate in training sessions as needed.

4. Knowledge of Camp Health Regulations: Research the specific regulations and guidelines related to camp nursing in your region or the area

where you plan to work. These may include state health department regulations, licensing requirements, and accreditation standards for camp healthcare services.

It's important to note that camp nursing positions are often seasonal and may require living on-site during the camp season. Be prepared for the unique challenges and rewards of working in a camp setting, providing healthcare services to campers and supporting their overall camp experience.

| Health Policy Nursing |

Health Policy Nursing is a specialty that focuses on the intersection of healthcare and public policy. Health Policy Nurses play a crucial role in shaping and advocating for policies that promote equitable access to healthcare, improve population health outcomes, and address healthcare system challenges. They work in various settings, including government agencies, advocacy organizations, research institutions, and healthcare organizations.

A Day in the Life

A typical day in the life of a Health Policy Nurse may involve:

1. Policy Research and Analysis: Conducting research on healthcare policies, legislation, and regulatory frameworks to understand their implications on nursing practice, healthcare delivery, and patient outcomes.

2. Policy Development and Advocacy: Participating in the development and implementation of healthcare policies, including drafting policy proposals, providing input on regulatory changes, and advocating for policy reforms that align with the interests of nursing professionals and the population's health needs.

3. Stakeholder Engagement: Collaborating with policymakers, healthcare professionals, patient advocacy groups, and other stakeholders to gather input, build consensus, and advocate for policies that address healthcare challenges and promote equitable healthcare access.

4. Data Collection and Analysis: Collecting and analyzing data on healthcare outcomes, disparities, and utilization patterns to inform policy recommendations and identify areas for improvement.

5. Policy Evaluation: Assessing the impact of healthcare policies on patient outcomes, healthcare delivery, and access to care, and providing evidence-based recommendations for policy modifications or interventions.

6. Communication and Education: Communicating policy recommendations to various stakeholders through written reports, presentations, and public speaking engagements. Educating nurses and healthcare professionals about policy issues, their implications, and opportunities for involvement.

7. Legislative and Regulatory Affairs: Monitoring and analyzing proposed legislation and regulations related to healthcare and nursing practice. Providing expert guidance on the potential impact of these policies and advocating for necessary amendments or revisions.

8. Collaborative Partnerships: Building and maintaining partnerships with government agencies, professional associations, research institutions, and community organizations to leverage collective expertise

and advance health policy initiatives.

9. Policy Implementation Support: Assisting healthcare organizations and institutions in implementing new policies and regulatory requirements, ensuring compliance, and promoting effective integration into practice.

10. Health Promotion and Education: Participating in health promotion campaigns, community outreach, and public education initiatives aimed at raising awareness of health policy issues and promoting public engagement in the policy-making process.

Degree(s) Required

To pursue a career in Health Policy Nursing, a minimum of a Bachelor of Science in Nursing (BSN) degree is typically required. However, many positions may prefer or require a Master of Science in Nursing (MSN) or a graduate degree in Health Policy, Public Health, or a related field. Advanced degrees provide a deeper understanding of health policy, research methods, and advocacy strategies.

Salary
$61,700 - $91,800

Specialty Certifications Available or Needed

While there are no specific certifications for Health Policy Nursing, obtaining certifications related to policy and advocacy can enhance your expertise and credibility in the field. Consider certifications such as:

1. Public Health Certification: The National Board of Public Health Examiners offers the Certified in Public Health (CPH) credential, which demonstrates knowledge and competency in public health principles, practices, and policies.

2. Health Policy Certifications: Various organizations, such as the American Association of Nurse Practitioners (AANP) and the American College of Healthcare Executives (ACHE), offer certifications or advanced degrees focused on health policy and management.

It's important to research and identify certifications that align with your career goals and the specific area of health policy you wish to specialize in.

Job Requirements

To work in Health Policy Nursing, consider the following job requirements:

1. Policy and Advocacy Knowledge: Deep understanding of healthcare policy issues, legislative processes, regulatory frameworks, and the ability to analyze policy implications on nursing practice, healthcare delivery, and population health.

2. Research and Analytical Skills: Proficiency in research methodologies, data analysis, and critical appraisal of evidence to inform policy development, evaluation, and recommendations.

3. Communication and Influencing Skills: Effective written and verbal communication skills to convey complex policy concepts to various audiences and engage in persuasive advocacy.

4. Collaboration and Networking: Ability to collaborate with diverse stakeholders, build relationships, and form alliances to advance health policy goals.

5. Policy Analysis and Evaluation: Experience in analyzing healthcare policies, assessing their impact, and providing evidence-based recommendations for policy improvements or modifications.

6. Political Acumen: Understanding the political landscape and navigating complex systems to advocate for policies that address health disparities, promote social justice, and enhance healthcare access.

7. Leadership and Project Management: Strong leadership skills to lead policy initiatives, manage projects, and coordinate multi-disciplinary teams working towards policy objectives.

8. Continuous Learning: Commitment to staying updated with emerging health policy trends, research, and legislation through ongoing professional development, conferences, and involvement in relevant policy organizations.

Miscellaneous Information You Should Know

To enter the field of Health Policy Nursing, consider the following:

1. Gain Policy Experience: Seek opportunities to gain policy-related experience, such as internships, fellowships, or volunteer work with government agencies, healthcare organizations, or policy research institutions.

2. Expand Your Knowledge: Stay informed about current policy issues and debates by reading policy journals, attending policy-focused conferences, and participating in policy forums or discussions.

3. Professional Engagement: Join professional organizations focused on health policy, public health, or nursing advocacy to network with professionals in the field, access resources, and stay connected with policy developments.

4. Advanced Education: Consider pursuing a graduate degree or

specialized training in Health Policy, Public Health, or a related field to gain in-depth knowledge and skills in policy analysis, research, and advocacy.

Working in Health Policy Nursing provides an opportunity to contribute to the development, implementation, and evaluation of policies that shape the healthcare landscape. It requires a solid understanding of healthcare policy issues, research methodologies, and effective advocacy strategies.

PART IV:

ADVANCED PRACTICE SPECIALTIES

| Family Nurse Practitioner (FNP) |

Family Nurse Practitioners (FNPs) are advanced practice registered nurses who provide comprehensive healthcare services to individuals and families across the lifespan. They are trained to diagnose and treat acute and chronic illnesses, promote health and wellness, and manage patients' overall healthcare needs. FNPs work in various settings, including primary care clinics, community health centers, urgent care facilities, and private practices, delivering patient-centered care with a focus on preventive care, health education, and disease management.

A Day in the Life

A day in the life of a Family Nurse Practitioner may involve the following activities:

1. Patient Assessment: Conducting comprehensive health assessments, including physical examinations, medical history reviews, and ordering diagnostic tests when necessary.

2. Diagnosis and Treatment: Diagnosing and treating acute illnesses, managing chronic conditions, prescribing medications, and developing care plans tailored to each patient's needs.

3. Health Promotion and Education: Providing health education and counseling on topics such as disease prevention, healthy lifestyle choices, and management of chronic conditions.

4. Preventive Care: Conducting screenings, immunizations, and preventive health interventions to promote wellness and identify early signs of disease.

5. Collaborative Care: Collaborating with healthcare teams, including physicians, specialists, and other healthcare professionals, to ensure coordinated and comprehensive care for patients.

6. Patient Advocacy: Advocating for patients' needs, rights, and access to quality healthcare services, including referrals to specialists or community resources.

7. Chronic Disease Management: Monitoring and managing chronic conditions such as diabetes, hypertension, asthma, and coordinating ongoing care to optimize patients' health outcomes.

8. Follow-up Care: Conducting routine follow-up visits, evaluating treatment effectiveness, adjusting care plans, and addressing any concerns or questions.

9. Health Record Documentation: Documenting patient encounters, treatment plans, and clinical findings in electronic health records (EHR) to maintain accurate and up-to-date patient information.

10. Collaborative Practice: Collaborating with other healthcare

professionals to develop and implement evidence-based practice guidelines and quality improvement initiatives.

Degree(s) Required

To become a Family Nurse Practitioner, the following degree(s) are typically required:

1. Bachelor of Science in Nursing (BSN): Obtain a BSN degree from an accredited nursing program, which typically takes four years to complete.

2. Master of Science in Nursing (MSN): Pursue an MSN degree with a specialization in Family Nurse Practitioner. The MSN program can take an additional two to three years to complete for registered nurses holding a BSN.

3. Doctor of Nursing Practice (DNP): Some individuals may choose to pursue a DNP degree, which provides advanced clinical and leadership training. The DNP program typically takes three to four years to complete after obtaining an MSN.

Salary

$95,090 - $120,340

Specialty Certifications Available or Needed

To practice as a Family Nurse Practitioner, certification through a national certifying body is required. Some recognized certifications for FNPs include:

1. American Academy of Nurse Practitioners Certification Board (AANPCB): Family Nurse Practitioner-Certified (FNP-C)

2. American Nurses Credentialing Center (ANCC): Family Nurse Practitioner-Board Certified (FNP-BC)

These certifications validate the nurse's advanced knowledge and clinical competence as a Family Nurse Practitioner.

Job Requirements

To work as a Family Nurse Practitioner, consider the following job requirements:

1. Licensure: Obtain a registered nurse (RN) license from the state where you plan to practice. Requirements may vary by state, so ensure compliance with the respective state board of nursing.

2. Certification: Obtain national certification as a Family Nurse Practitioner through AANPCB or ANCC.

3. Clinical Experience: Gain relevant clinical experience as a registered nurse, preferably in primary care or a related field, to develop a strong foundation in patient care and assessment.

4. Advanced Practice Registered Nurse (APRN) Recognition: In some states, APRN recognition is required in addition to RN licensure. This recognition grants authority to practice as an advanced practice nurse, including prescribing medications and ordering diagnostic tests.

5. Collaborative Practice Agreement: Some states require a collaborative practice agreement with a supervising physician, outlining the scope of practice and collaborative relationship.

6. Continuing Education: Maintain ongoing professional development by attending conferences, workshops, and continuing education programs to stay updated on the latest research, guidelines, and advancements in primary care.

Miscellaneous Information You Should Know

Consider the following miscellaneous information to enter the Family Nurse Practitioner specialty:

1. Certification Maintenance: Certification as a Family Nurse Practitioner requires periodic renewal through continuing education and meeting the certification board's requirements.

2. Professional Associations: Consider joining professional associations such as the American Association of Nurse Practitioners (AANP) or the National Association of Pediatric Nurse Practitioners (NAPNAP) to access resources, networking opportunities, and advocacy efforts specific to the FNP specialty.

3. State Practice Regulations: Familiarize yourself with the regulations and practice requirements specific to the state(s) where you plan to practice as an FNP, as regulations may vary regarding scope of practice, prescriptive authority, and collaborative agreements.

Becoming a Family Nurse Practitioner offers the opportunity to provide comprehensive primary care, improve health outcomes, and establish long-term relationships with patients and their families. It requires advanced education, clinical experience, ongoing professional development, and a passion for delivering holistic, patient-centered care.

| Certified Registered Nurse Anesthetist (CRNA) |

Certified Registered Nurse Anesthetists (CRNAs) are advanced practice registered nurses who specialize in providing anesthesia and pain management services to patients across various healthcare settings. They work in collaboration with surgeons, anesthesiologists, and other healthcare professionals to administer anesthesia during surgical procedures, monitor patients' vital signs, manage pain, and ensure safe anesthesia outcomes. CRNAs are responsible for assessing patients' pre-operative conditions, selecting appropriate anesthesia techniques, administering anesthesia, and providing post-operative care.

A Day in the Life

A day in the life of a CRNA may involve the following activities:

1. Patient Assessment: Conducting thorough pre-operative assessments, including reviewing medical history, performing physical examinations, and evaluating patients' readiness for anesthesia.

2. Anesthesia Planning: Collaborating with the surgical team to develop an individualized anesthesia plan based on the patient's medical condition, type of surgery, and expected outcomes.

3. Anesthesia Administration: Administering various types of anesthesia, such as general anesthesia, regional anesthesia, or sedation, using advanced techniques and monitoring equipment to ensure patient comfort and safety during surgery.

4. Intraoperative Monitoring: Continuously monitoring patients' vital signs, including heart rate, blood pressure, oxygen saturation, and anesthesia depth, adjusting anesthesia levels as needed throughout the procedure.

5. Patient Safety: Ensuring the patient's safety and well-being during the surgery, including managing airway, fluid status, and pain control.

6. Emergency Response: Being prepared to handle any anesthesia-related emergencies that may arise during the procedure, such as adverse reactions or complications.

7. Post-Anesthesia Care: Providing post-anesthetic care, monitoring patients in the recovery room, and managing pain and nausea.

8. Collaboration and Communication: Collaborating with the surgical team, anesthesiologists, and other healthcare professionals to ensure seamless patient care and effective communication throughout the perioperative period.

9. Continuing Education: Staying updated on the latest advancements in anesthesia techniques, medications, and patient safety

protocols through ongoing professional development and continuing education.

Degree(s) Required

To become a Certified Registered Nurse Anesthetist (CRNA), the following degree(s) are typically required:

1. Bachelor of Science in Nursing (BSN): Obtain a BSN degree from an accredited nursing program, which typically takes four years to complete.
2. Registered Nurse (RN) Licensure: Obtain a registered nurse (RN) license by passing the National Council Licensure Examination for Registered Nurses (NCLEX-RN).
3. Master of Science in Nursing (MSN) in Nurse Anesthesia: Pursue an accredited MSN program with a specialization in Nurse Anesthesia. The MSN program typically takes an additional two to three years to complete for registered nurses holding a BSN.
4. Doctor of Nursing Practice (DNP): Some CRNA programs may require or offer the option to pursue a Doctor of Nursing Practice (DNP) degree. The DNP program provides additional advanced training and may take an additional one to two years to complete.

Salary

$160,030 - $200,640

Specialty Certifications Available or Needed

To practice as a CRNA, certification through the National Board of Certification and Recertification for Nurse Anesthetists (NBCRNA) is required. The certification is known as the National Certification Examination for Nurse Anesthetists (NCE). Passing this exam is necessary to become a certified CRNA.

Job Requirements

To work as a CRNA, consider the following job requirements:

1. Licensure: Obtain a registered nurse (RN) license from the state where you plan to practice. Requirements may vary by state, so ensure compliance with the respective state board of nursing.
2. Graduate Education: Complete an accredited MSN or DNP program with a specialization in Nurse Anesthesia.
3. Clinical Experience: Acquire a significant amount of clinical experience in critical care nursing, as most CRNA programs require a minimum of one to two years of experience in an acute care setting.

4. Certification: Pass the National Certification Examination for Nurse Anesthetists (NCE) administered by the NBCRNA.

5. State Practice Regulations: Familiarize yourself with state-specific regulations and requirements for CRNAs, including prescriptive authority, scope of practice, and collaborative agreements if applicable.

6. Continuing Education: Maintain ongoing professional development and fulfill continuing education requirements to maintain certification and stay updated on the latest advances in anesthesia practice.

Miscellaneous Information You Should Know

Consider the following miscellaneous information to enter the CRNA specialty:

1. Competency and Skills: CRNAs require a high level of technical skills, critical thinking, and decision-making abilities. Attention to detail, excellent communication skills, and the ability to work well under pressure are essential.

2. On-call and Flexible Schedule: CRNAs may work on-call or have irregular work hours, including nights, weekends, and holidays, depending on the healthcare setting and patient needs.

3. Professional Organizations: Consider joining professional organizations such as the American Association of Nurse Anesthetists (AANA) to access resources, continuing education opportunities, networking, and advocacy efforts specific to the CRNA specialty.

Becoming a Certified Registered Nurse Anesthetist requires advanced education, clinical experience, and the ability to provide safe and effective anesthesia care to patients. CRNAs play a critical role in the surgical team, ensuring patient comfort and safety throughout the perioperative period.

| Nurse Midwife |

Nurse Midwives are advanced practice registered nurses who specialize in providing comprehensive healthcare to women throughout their lifespan, with a focus on pregnancy, childbirth, and postpartum care. They provide a wide range of services, including prenatal care, labor and delivery support, postpartum care, family planning, gynecological exams, and primary healthcare for women. Nurse Midwives emphasize the promotion of holistic and individualized care, empowering women to actively participate in their healthcare decisions.

A Day in the Life

A day in the life of a Nurse Midwife may involve the following activities:

1. Prenatal Care: Conducting prenatal examinations, including assessing the health of the mother and baby, monitoring fetal development, providing education and counseling on pregnancy, and addressing any concerns or complications.

2. Labor and Delivery: Providing support and guidance to women during labor and delivery, assisting with pain management techniques, monitoring the progress of labor, and facilitating a safe and positive birth experience.

3. Postpartum Care: Conducting postpartum assessments, providing care for the mother and newborn, assisting with breastfeeding support, offering guidance on newborn care and parenting, and addressing any postpartum complications or concerns.

4. Family Planning and Reproductive Health: Providing contraception counseling, performing gynecological exams, offering family planning services, including prescribing and fitting contraceptive methods, and addressing reproductive health concerns.

5. Well-Woman Care: Conducting routine gynecological exams, including Pap smears, breast exams, and screenings for sexually transmitted infections, and addressing women's health concerns and preventive care.

6. Education and Counseling: Providing patient education on various topics, including pregnancy, childbirth, breastfeeding, contraception, sexual health, and menopause, empowering women to make informed decisions about their health.

7. Collaboration and Referrals: Collaborating with other healthcare professionals, such as obstetricians, pediatricians, and primary care providers, and making referrals as needed for specialized care.

8. Documentation and Record-Keeping: Maintaining accurate and up-to-date patient records, documenting assessments, interventions, and

care plans, and ensuring compliance with legal and regulatory requirements.

Degree(s) Required

To become a Nurse Midwife, the following degree(s) are typically required:

1. Bachelor of Science in Nursing (BSN): Obtain a BSN degree from an accredited nursing program, which typically takes four years to complete.

2. Registered Nurse (RN) Licensure: Obtain a registered nurse (RN) license by passing the National Council Licensure Examination for Registered Nurses (NCLEX-RN).

3. Master of Science in Nursing (MSN) in Nurse Midwifery: Pursue an accredited MSN program with a specialization in Nurse Midwifery. The MSN program typically takes an additional two to three years to complete for registered nurses holding a BSN.

Salary

$90,410 - $148,260

Specialty Certifications Available or Needed

To practice as a Nurse Midwife, certification through the American Midwifery Certification Board (AMCB) is typically required. The certification is known as the Certified Nurse Midwife (CNM). Passing the AMCB examination is necessary to become a certified Nurse Midwife.

Job Requirements

To work as a Nurse Midwife, consider the following job requirements:

1. Licensure: Obtain a registered nurse (RN) license from the state where you plan to practice. Requirements may vary by state, so ensure compliance with the respective state board of nursing.

2. Graduate Education: Complete an accredited MSN program with a specialization in Nurse Midwifery.

3. Clinical Experience: Acquire a significant amount of clinical experience in women's health, including prenatal care, labor and delivery, and postpartum care. Most MSN programs require a minimum number of hours of clinical experience.

4. Certification: Pass the Certified Nurse Midwife (CNM) examination administered by the American Midwifery Certification Board (AMCB).

5. State Practice Regulations: Familiarize yourself with state-specific

regulations and requirements for Nurse Midwives, including scope of practice, prescriptive authority, collaborative agreements, and licensure renewal.

Miscellaneous Information You Should Know

Consider the following miscellaneous information to enter the Nurse Midwife specialty:

1. Compassion and Empathy: Nurse Midwives should possess excellent interpersonal skills, empathy, and the ability to provide emotional support to women and their families during the childbirth process.

2. Commitment to Women's Health: A passion for women's health, including reproductive health, family planning, and providing comprehensive care throughout a woman's lifespan.

3. Collaboration and Communication: Nurse Midwives work closely with other healthcare professionals, including obstetricians, pediatricians, and primary care providers, requiring effective collaboration and communication skills.

4. Continuing Education: Maintaining ongoing professional development and fulfilling continuing education requirements to stay updated on the latest evidence-based practices and advancements in women's health and midwifery care.

Becoming a Nurse Midwife requires advanced education, clinical experience, and a commitment to providing comprehensive and holistic care to women throughout their lifespan. Nurse Midwives play a crucial role in promoting and supporting healthy pregnancies, childbirth experiences, and women's overall well-being.

| Adult-Gerontology Nurse Practitioner (AGNP) |

Adult-Gerontology Nurse Practitioners (AGNPs) are advanced practice registered nurses who specialize in providing comprehensive healthcare to adult and older adult populations. They are trained to assess, diagnose, and manage common acute and chronic illnesses, promote health and wellness, and provide holistic care to individuals across the adult lifespan. AGNPs may work in a variety of settings, including primary care clinics, specialty clinics, hospitals, long-term care facilities, and home healthcare.

A Day in the Life

A day in the life of an Adult-Gerontology Nurse Practitioner may involve the following activities:

1. Patient Assessments: Conducting comprehensive health assessments, including physical examinations, medical history reviews, and assessment of current symptoms or concerns.

2. Diagnosis and Treatment: Ordering and interpreting diagnostic tests, formulating differential diagnoses, developing treatment plans, prescribing medications, and providing patient education.

3. Chronic Disease Management: Managing chronic conditions such as diabetes, hypertension, heart disease, and respiratory disorders, including monitoring patients' health status, adjusting medications, and providing counseling on lifestyle modifications.

4. Acute Care: Diagnosing and treating acute illnesses and injuries, such as infections, injuries, and respiratory conditions, and coordinating appropriate follow-up care.

5. Health Promotion and Preventive Care: Promoting health and wellness through preventive screenings, immunizations, health counseling, and lifestyle interventions.

6. Collaboration and Referrals: Collaborating with other healthcare professionals, such as specialists, pharmacists, and physical therapists, and making referrals for specialized care when necessary.

7. Patient Education: Providing patient education on disease management, medication adherence, lifestyle modifications, and self-care strategies.

8. Follow-up and Continuity of Care: Conducting follow-up visits to monitor patients' progress, adjust treatment plans, and ensure continuity of care.

Degree(s) Required

To become an Adult-Gerontology Nurse Practitioner, the

following degree(s) are typically required:

1. Bachelor of Science in Nursing (BSN): Obtain a BSN degree from an accredited nursing program, which typically takes four years to complete.
2. Registered Nurse (RN) Licensure: Obtain a registered nurse (RN) license by passing the National Council Licensure Examination for Registered Nurses (NCLEX-RN).
3. Master of Science in Nursing (MSN) or Doctor of Nursing Practice (DNP) in Adult-Gerontology: Pursue an accredited MSN or DNP program with a specialization in Adult-Gerontology. The program typically takes an additional two to three years to complete for registered nurses holding a BSN.

Salary
$95,000 - $124,820

Specialty Certifications Available or Needed
To practice as an Adult-Gerontology Nurse Practitioner, certification through a recognized certification body is typically required. Some certification options include:

1. American Nurses Credentialing Center (ANCC): Adult-Gerontology Primary Care Nurse Practitioner Certification (AGPCNP-BC)

2. American Association of Nurse Practitioners (AANP): Adult-Gerontology Primary Care Nurse Practitioner Certification (AGPCNP-BC)

Certification demonstrates a nurse practitioner's expertise and competence in the Adult-Gerontology specialty.

Job Requirements
To work as an Adult-Gerontology Nurse Practitioner, consider the following job requirements:

1. Licensure: Obtain an advanced practice registered nurse (APRN) license from the state where you plan to practice. APRN licensure typically requires an active RN license and completion of an accredited AGNP program.
2. Graduate Education: Complete an accredited MSN or DNP program with a specialization in Adult-Gerontology.
3. Clinical Experience: Acquire a significant amount of clinical experience caring for adult and older adult populations across various

healthcare settings, including primary care and specialty clinics.

4. Certification: Pass the certification examination specific to Adult-Gerontology offered by recognized certification bodies such as ANCC or AANP.

5. State Practice Regulations: Familiarize yourself with state-specific regulations and requirements for Adult-Gerontology Nurse Practitioners, including scope of practice, prescriptive authority, collaborative agreements, and licensure renewal.

Miscellaneous Information You Should Know

Consider the following miscellaneous information to enter the Adult-Gerontology Nurse Practitioner specialty:

1. Communication and Interpersonal Skills: AGNPs must have excellent communication skills to establish rapport with patients, collaborate with healthcare teams, and educate individuals on healthcare management.

2. Gerontological Competencies: A strong understanding of gerontology, including age-related changes, common health conditions, and management strategies specific to the older adult population.

3. Lifelong Learning: Commitment to ongoing professional development to stay updated on the latest evidence-based practices, guidelines, and advancements in the field of adult and gerontological healthcare.

4. Cultural Competence: Sensitivity to diverse cultural backgrounds and the ability to provide culturally appropriate care to individuals from various ethnic, religious, and socioeconomic backgrounds.

Becoming an Adult-Gerontology Nurse Practitioner requires advanced education, clinical experience, and a commitment to providing comprehensive and patient-centered care to adult and older adult populations. AGNPs play a vital role in promoting health, managing chronic conditions, and improving the quality of life for individuals across the adult lifespan.

| Psychiatric Mental Health Nurse Practitioner (PMHNP) |

Psychiatric Mental Health Nurse Practitioners (PMHNPs) are advanced practice registered nurses who specialize in providing mental health care to individuals across the lifespan. They assess, diagnose, and manage psychiatric disorders, provide therapy and counseling, prescribe medications, and promote mental wellness. PMHNPs work in various healthcare settings, including psychiatric hospitals, mental health clinics, community health centers, and private practices.

A Day in the Life

A day in the life of a Psychiatric Mental Health Nurse Practitioner may involve the following activities:

1. Patient Assessments: Conducting comprehensive psychiatric evaluations, including mental health history, symptom assessments, and risk assessments.

2. Diagnosis and Treatment: Diagnosing and treating mental health disorders, including mood disorders, anxiety disorders, psychotic disorders, and substance use disorders. Developing treatment plans, prescribing appropriate medications, and providing psychotherapy and counseling.

3. Medication Management: Monitoring medication effectiveness, adjusting dosages as needed, and educating patients about the benefits and potential side effects of medications.

4. Psychotherapy and Counseling: Providing individual and group therapy sessions, counseling patients on coping strategies, stress management, and lifestyle changes to improve mental well-being.

5. Crisis Intervention: Responding to mental health crises, assessing for suicide risk, and coordinating emergency interventions when necessary.

6. Collaboration and Referrals: Collaborating with other healthcare professionals, such as psychologists, social workers, and psychiatrists, to provide comprehensive care. Making referrals for specialized services when needed.

7. Patient Education: Educating patients and their families about mental health conditions, treatment options, self-care techniques, and community resources.

8. Follow-up and Continuity of Care: Conducting follow-up visits to monitor patients' progress, adjust treatment plans, and ensure continuity of care.

Degree(s) Required

To become a Psychiatric Mental Health Nurse Practitioner, the following degree(s) are typically required:

1. Bachelor of Science in Nursing (BSN): Obtain a BSN degree from an accredited nursing program, which typically takes four years to complete.
2. Registered Nurse (RN) Licensure: Obtain a registered nurse (RN) license by passing the National Council Licensure Examination for Registered Nurses (NCLEX-RN).
3. Master of Science in Nursing (MSN) or Doctor of Nursing Practice (DNP) in Psychiatric Mental Health: Pursue an accredited MSN or DNP program with a specialization in Psychiatric Mental Health. The program typically takes an additional two to three years to complete for registered nurses holding a BSN.

Salary
$110,740 - $198,320

Specialty Certifications Available or Needed
Certification in Psychiatric Mental Health Nursing is available for PMHNPs. The primary certification bodies offering specialty certifications include:

1. American Nurses Credentialing Center (ANCC): Psychiatric-Mental Health Nurse Practitioner Certification (PMHNP-BC)

2. American Association of Nurse Practitioners (AANP): Psychiatric-Mental Health Nurse Practitioner Certification (PMHNP-BC)

Certification demonstrates competence in the field and may be required or preferred by employers.

Job Requirements
To work as a Psychiatric Mental Health Nurse Practitioner, consider the following job requirements:

1. Licensure: Obtain an advanced practice registered nurse (APRN) license from the state where you plan to practice. APRN licensure typically requires an active RN license and completion of an accredited PMHNP program.
2. Graduate Education: Complete an accredited MSN or DNP program with a specialization in Psychiatric Mental Health.
3. Clinical Experience: Acquire a significant amount of clinical

experience in psychiatric and mental health settings, including assessment, diagnosis, and management of mental health disorders.

4. Certification: Pass the certification examination specific to Psychiatric Mental Health offered by recognized certification bodies such as ANCC or AANP.

5. State Practice Regulations: Familiarize yourself with state-specific regulations and requirements for PMHNPs, including scope of practice, prescriptive authority, collaborative agreements, and licensure renewal.

Miscellaneous Information You Should Know

Consider the following miscellaneous information to enter the Psychiatric Mental Health Nurse Practitioner specialty:

1. Strong Interpersonal and Communication Skills: PMHNPs need excellent communication and interpersonal skills to establish rapport with patients, conduct thorough assessments, and provide compassionate care.

2. Non-Judgmental Attitude: Being non-judgmental and open-minded is crucial to creating a safe and supportive environment for patients with mental health concerns.

3. Cultural Competence: Sensitivity to diverse cultural backgrounds and the ability to provide culturally appropriate care to individuals from various ethnic, religious, and socioeconomic backgrounds.

4. Commitment to Lifelong Learning: Stay updated on the latest research, treatment modalities, and evidence-based practices in psychiatric and mental health care through continuing education and professional development opportunities.

Becoming a Psychiatric Mental Health Nurse Practitioner requires advanced education, clinical experience, and a passion for providing holistic mental health care to individuals across the lifespan. PMHNPs play a vital role in promoting mental well-being and improving the overall quality of life for their patients.

| Clinical Nurse Specialist |

Clinical Nurse Specialists (CNS) are advanced practice registered nurses who specialize in a specific patient population, clinical setting, or health condition. They provide expert clinical knowledge, leadership, and direct patient care. CNSs work in various healthcare settings, including hospitals, clinics, research institutions, and educational facilities. They are instrumental in improving patient outcomes, influencing healthcare policies, and implementing evidence-based practices.

A Day in the Life

A day in the life of a Clinical Nurse Specialist may involve the following activities:

1. Patient Assessment and Diagnosis: Conducting comprehensive patient assessments, including physical examinations, medical histories, and diagnostic tests, to determine patient needs, identify health problems, and develop appropriate care plans.

2. Direct Patient Care: Providing direct patient care, including administering treatments, managing complex medical conditions, monitoring patient progress, and coordinating care among healthcare providers.

3. Education and Counseling: Educating patients, families, and healthcare staff on disease management, treatment options, preventive care, and health promotion strategies.

4. Leadership and Consultation: Collaborating with interdisciplinary healthcare teams, providing clinical leadership, and acting as a resource for nurses, physicians, and other healthcare professionals.

5. Research and Evidence-Based Practice: Participating in research initiatives, implementing evidence-based practices, and evaluating the effectiveness of healthcare interventions to improve patient outcomes.

6. Quality Improvement: Identifying areas for improvement in patient care, developing quality improvement initiatives, and monitoring performance indicators to enhance healthcare delivery and patient safety.

7. Policy and Advocacy: Contributing to healthcare policy development, advocating for patients and their families, and influencing healthcare practices at the organizational and system levels.

8. Professional Development: Engaging in continuous learning, attending conferences, staying updated on advancements in healthcare, and participating in professional organizations and committees.

Degree(s) Required

To become a Clinical Nurse Specialist, the following degree(s) are typically required:

1. Bachelor of Science in Nursing (BSN): Obtain a BSN degree from an accredited nursing program, which typically takes four years to complete.
2. Registered Nurse (RN) Licensure: Obtain a registered nurse (RN) license by passing the National Council Licensure Examination for Registered Nurses (NCLEX-RN).
3. Master of Science in Nursing (MSN) or Doctor of Nursing Practice (DNP) with a Clinical Nurse Specialist specialization: Pursue an accredited MSN or DNP program with a concentration in Clinical Nurse Specialist. The program generally takes an additional two to three years to complete for registered nurses holding a BSN.

Salary
$91,120 - $122,540

Specialty Certifications Available or Needed
Certification as a Clinical Nurse Specialist is available to validate expertise in the specialty. The certification is typically offered by professional nursing organizations such as:

1. American Nurses Credentialing Center (ANCC): Clinical Nurse Specialist Certification (CNS-BC)

2. American Association of Critical-Care Nurses (AACN): Acute Care Clinical Nurse Specialist Certification (ACNS-BC)

Certification demonstrates advanced knowledge and competencies in the specialty area.

Job Requirements
To work as a Clinical Nurse Specialist, consider the following job requirements:

1. Licensure: Obtain an advanced practice registered nurse (APRN) license from the state where you plan to practice. APRN licensure typically requires an active RN license and completion of an accredited CNS program.
2. Graduate Education: Complete an accredited MSN or DNP program with a specialization in Clinical Nurse Specialist.
3. Clinical Experience: Acquire a significant amount of clinical experience in the chosen specialty area, demonstrating advanced skills and

knowledge.

4. Certification: Pass the certification examination specific to Clinical Nurse Specialist offered by recognized certification bodies such as ANCC or AACN.

5. State Practice Regulations: Familiarize yourself with state-specific regulations and requirements for CNSs, including scope of practice, prescriptive authority, collaborative agreements, and licensure renewal.

Miscellaneous Information You Should Know

Consider the following miscellaneous information to enter the Clinical Nurse Specialist specialty:

1. Strong Clinical Expertise: CNSs should possess in-depth knowledge and expertise in their chosen specialty area to provide specialized care, education, and consultation.

2. Leadership Skills: Strong leadership and communication skills are essential for collaborating with healthcare teams, advocating for patients, and influencing practice changes.

3. Research and Analytical Skills: Proficiency in research methods, data analysis, and evidence-based practice is important for integrating research findings into clinical practice and driving quality improvement initiatives.

4. Lifelong Learning: A commitment to continuous learning and professional development is crucial to stay updated on advancements in the field, healthcare policy changes, and emerging best practices.

Becoming a Clinical Nurse Specialist requires advanced education, clinical experience, and a dedication to improving patient outcomes through specialized care, leadership, and evidence-based practice. CNSs play a vital role in enhancing healthcare delivery, promoting quality care, and serving as advocates for their patients and the nursing profession.

INDEX

ABOUT THE AUTHOR

Mitch LaFleur is an accomplished and highly skilled Registered Nurse with a passion for education, research, and leadership in the nursing progression and healthcare at large.

Education has been a cornerstone of Mitch's nursing journey, as evidenced by an impressive array of degrees earned and courses taught. Leveling up each of his educational qualifications, Mitch has seamlessly transitioned from the bedside (as an Emergency Department Nurse) to higher education.

He currently works as an Assistant Professor of Nursing at Georgian Court University, a small private university in New Jersey. His teaching philosophy focuses on bringing a sensible realism to the classroom, the goal of which is to impart valuable nursing insights that students will incorporate into their lifelong nursing practice. When not lecturing, Mitch serves as an Advising Fellow, helping to guide nursing students into a career path they love (which is how he got the idea for this book).

In addition to his teaching and advising duties, Mitch is actively involved in research endeavors and has a keen interest in exploring new horizons within the nursing field. His research interests include the utilization of Augmented Reality for Nursing Simulation Experiences, Nursing Mentorship Programs, and the examination of Stress & Burnout in Emergency Department Nurses. Through his research, Mitch seeks to enhance nursing practices, improve patient outcomes, and contribute to the advancement of the nursing profession.

When Mitch isn't busy making strides in the nursing world, he enjoys indulging in a few beloved hobbies. An ocean enthusiast at heart, he loves surfing and stand-up paddleboarding, finding solace in the embrace of the ocean. A bonified black coffee fanatic, Mitch will often be seen, on-campus or off, holding a cup of his favorite Hawaiian java. And perhaps most importantly, he cherishes quality time spent with his daughter; usually involving outdoor activities and coastal exploration in their Ford Transit Van.

THANK YOU

I extend my sincerest gratitude for choosing to embark on this nursing specialty-finding exploration with me. Your support and readership are so appreciated. Here's to having unbridled success at every stop on your nursing adventure!

- Mitch

Made in United States
Cleveland, OH
25 October 2024

10309788R00167